Foreword

As I was reviewing this book I saw a programme on television featuring a man who could stretch his skin anywhere on his body. It was fascinating and it made me think about how we take our skin for granted and why we need to look after it.

This excellent book by Dr John Gray is the sister book to *The World of Hair* and is similarly full of absorbing knowledge, facts and myths.

If you are studying for qualifications, working in the beauty industry, researching data or just fascinated with the concept of healthy skin, make sure you invest the time to read this book.

ALAN GOLDSBRO
Chief Executive
The Beauty Industry Authority

THE BEAUTY INDUSTRY
AUTHORITY

THE WORLD OF
SKIN CARE

A Scientific Companion

Dʀ JOHN GRAY

Contributors

Dr C. L. Gummer
Senior Research Fellow P&G

Dr P. J. Matts
Principal Scientist P&G

Professor R. Marks
Emeritus Professor of Dermatology, Universities of Wales and Miami

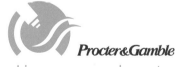

Procter&Gamble
skincare research centre

in association with the
Beauty Industry Authority

First published 2000 by
MACMILLAN PRESS LTD
Houndmills, Basingstoke, Hampshire RG21 6XS
and London
Companies and representatives
throughout the world

ISBN 0–333–77493–0

A catalogue record for this book is available
from the British Library.

This book is printed on paper suitable for recycling and
made from fully managed and sustained forest sources.

10   9   8   7   6   5   4   3   2   1
09 08 07 06 05 04 03 02 01 00

Printed in Great Britain by
Jarrold Book Printing, Thetford, Norfolk

The author

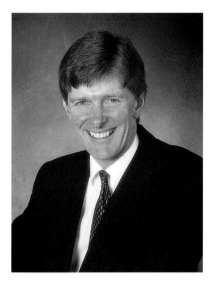

Dr John Gray is a partner in a large group practice and has a long-standing interest in skin and hair problems. He is a Consultant to Procter & Gamble at their UK research centre. He has written and lectured widely on the subject of cosmetic products and their benefits.

He is an elected member of the European and American Hair Research Societies, the Royal Society of Medicine and the European Society of Contact Dermatitis.

The contributors

Dr Christopher Gummer gained his doctorate at Oxford studying genetic and acquired hair diseases. He is currently the Senior Research Fellow at Procter & Gamble, and is recognised internationally as a world-class specialist in cosmetics development, leading hair and skin research in Europe.

Dr Paul Matts graduated and gained his doctorate at the University of Cardiff. He is now a Principal Scientist at Procter & Gamble, specialising in research into skin physiology and the benefits of cosmetic products. He is a member of COLIPA (the European Cosmetic, Toiletry and Perfumery Association).

Professor Ronald Marks is Emeritus Professor in the University of Wales and a Clinical Professor in the University of Miami School of Medicine. He is based in the Skin Care Cardiff clinic in Cardiff, Wales, U.K. He has written extensively, and is the author/co-author of over 35 books and over 350 articles in scientific and medical journals. He has been the President of the European Society for Dermatological Research, and is Life President of the International Society of Bioengineering and the Skin and President of the British Cosmetic Dermatology Group.

Acknowledgements

My thanks are due to:

Dorte and Kristiana for their love and support and for teaching me, a mere male,
the truth about skin care and the use of cosmetics

Janet Smith, my long-suffering secretary, for all her hard work in organisation

Jean Macqueen, my most splendid editor

Margaret and all at Hair Collections Club, Weybridge

Inner Sanctum-Beauticians, Old Windsor

and all those colleagues, patients and folk in the streets of the world who
allowed me to photograph them.

*The author and publishers wish to thank
the following illustration sources:*

Department of Dermatology, Kings College Hospital p. 146
F8 Imaging p. 132
Professor Ronald Marks p. 65 (foot)
Hugh Rushton p. 30 (bottom left)
Sotheby's p. 133
Telegraph Colour Library p. 84

*'From fairest creature we desire increase that
thereby beauty's rose might never die'*

William Shakespeare

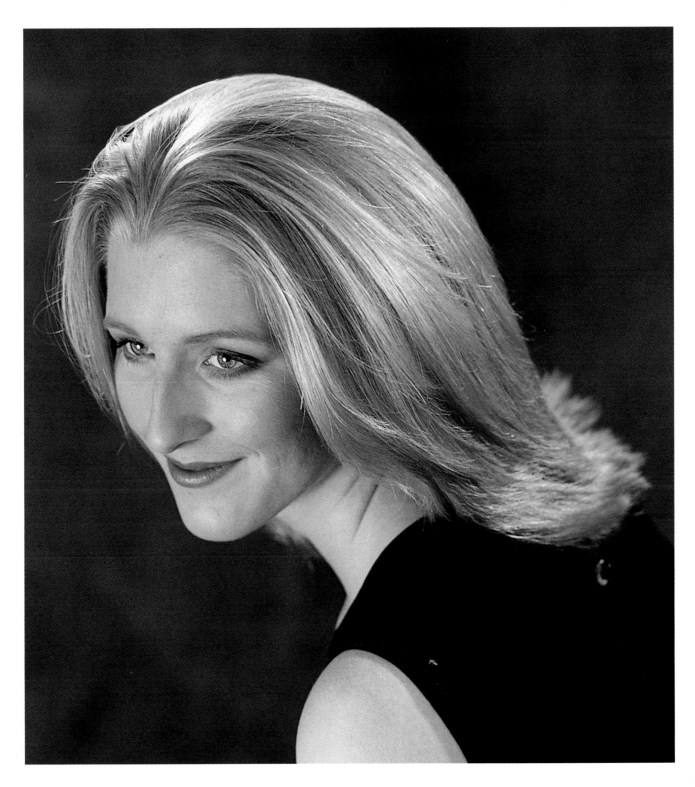

'...beauty's conquest of your face...'

W. H. Auden

Contents

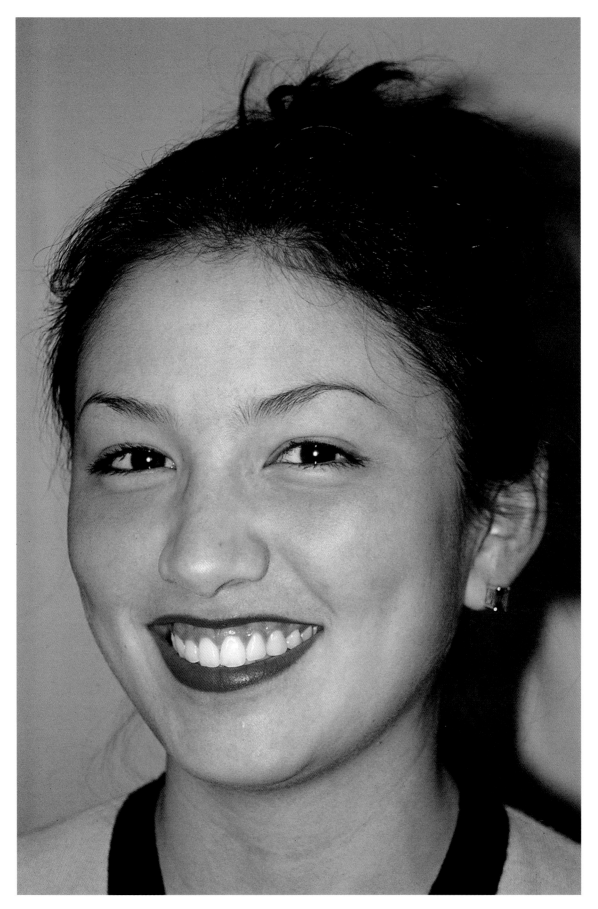

Maintaining beauty is a lifetime's task.

Introduction

Why another book on skin, and particularly on skin care? What is there to be said that is not already covered in the hundreds of magazine articles on beauty and skin health that are published every week?

Our skin is the outward appearance of who or what we are, or would like to be. But it is more than just a simple cover. It is the largest organ of the body – a complex and dynamic system that is vitally important to our health, and sometimes reflects it as well.

Every baby's skin, perhaps after a wrinkly start, looks very much like that of every other child within its racial group. But as the years go by its structure and appearance may change dramatically, and seldom for the better. Differences between the various parts of our skin, particularly that of sun-exposed areas like the face and arms, become more obvious.

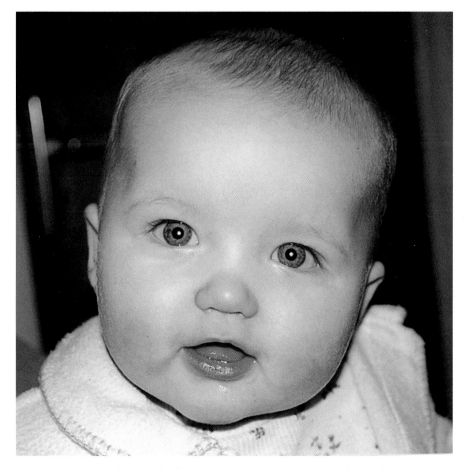

Skin usually gets off to a splendid start, without wrinkles, blemishes or furrows.

The changes that appear, and become more marked as the years go by, are a combination of natural ageing and damage from the sun's invisible rays.

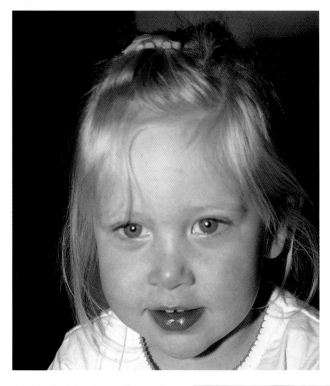

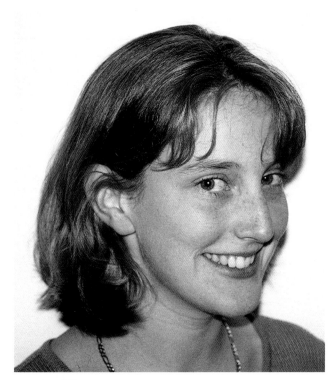

▲ *Skin that is still perfect and unblemished in the first decade of life.*

▲ *The third decade: beauty at the zenith of its powers.*

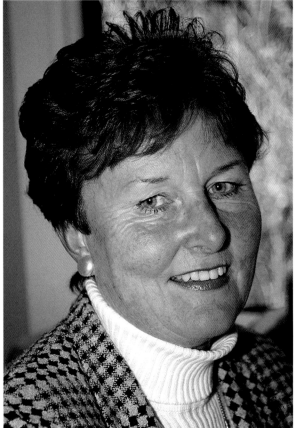

◄ *By the sixth decade we will all have visible changes to our skin, mostly due to earlier exposure to sunlight. This is when the benefits of regular skin care becomes more evident, as this elegant lady has found.*

A very few fortunate people hardly seem to age at all, and stay clear of serious wrinkles and blemishes well into old age.

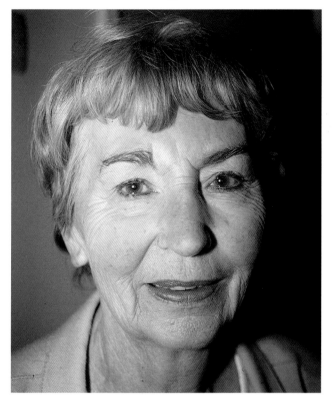

A lady who has cared for her beautiful skin for 75 years, but now is showing the inevitable signs of ageing.

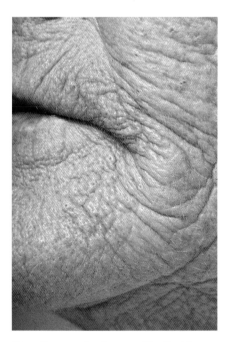

Deep furrows develop on skin that has experienced years of exposure to both sunlight and tobacco smoke.

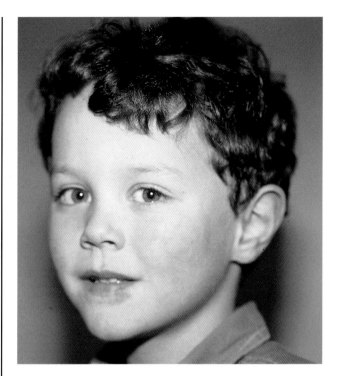

The 'bloom' of youth.

The skin of others, however, becomes so wrinkled and blotchy that they are almost unrecognisable to friends who have not seen them since their youth. How is this possible – what happened to their skin? And, more importantly, *why* do these changes happen?

What is the scientific explanation for the 'bloom of youth'? Why does an older person's skin naturally become drier? Why does the skin of some individuals seem to need little care, while other people spend much of their time and money trying to repair and disguise the effects of the passing years? Which, if any, among the thousands of alleged 'miracle' treatments claiming to make us look younger is worth buying and using? What, in short, is 'good' skin care?

This book is designed to bring to the reader the answers to some of these questions in terms of science behind what our skin is and does, and the products that can be used to 'preserve' or decorate it. It also aims to shed light on some common claims – and myths – that are put forward concerning skin care. It deals with ways of preventing damage and premature ageing of our skin, and describes how to make the best of what nature gave us through regularly using appropriate skin care routines and products from an early age.

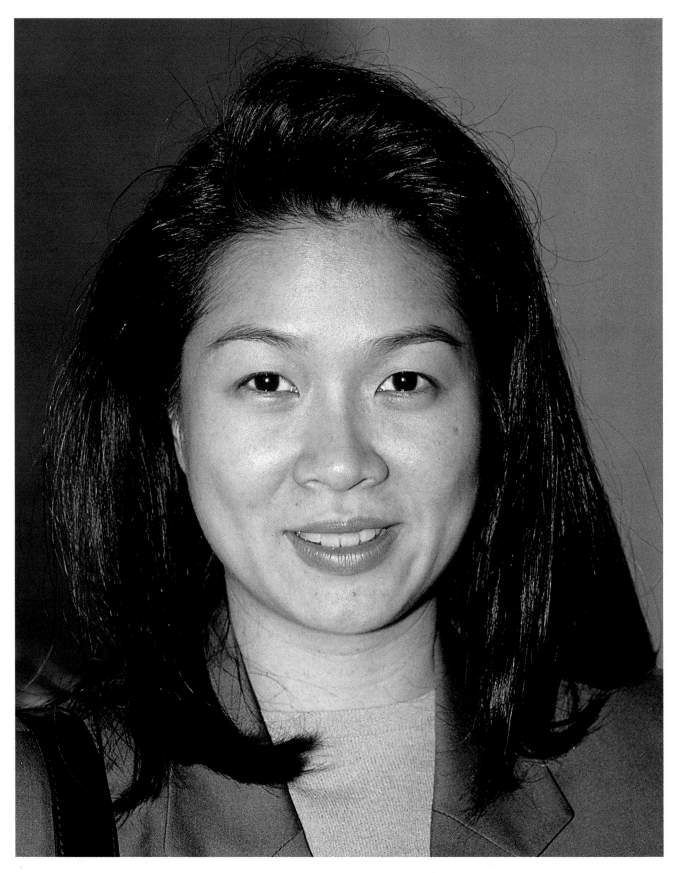

The skin is more than just a decorative covering; it is our living barrier to the outside world.

1
Skin structure

Look at your face in a mirror. What do you see?

At first sight your skin looks like a simple, decorative covering for your body, but it is far more than this. For instance, parts of it develop from the same tissues as the brain, and remain directly connected to the brain by nerves. Skin is a vital outpost of the nervous system and is the closest contact we have with the outside world. Our sense of touch operates through our skin: we feel pain and changes in temperature. The lips, which are part of the skin, are amongst the most sensitive areas of the body.

Skin is not just a simple flat sheet, but is composed of several layers. The very top layer is quite tough and, although microscopically thin, is our 'hide'. It is being constantly worn down and replaced. It plays a vital part in preventing excessive loss of moisture from the body, and helps to give healthy skin its attractive appearance. The deeper layers contain all the structures that give skin its strength and elasticity, and are home to important structures like the hair roots and sweat glands.

As we age the natural strength and elasticity in our skin declines, with the result that gravity makes it sag and wrinkles develop. Although certain skin care products make wild claims to be able to 'restore' youth, there is no evidence that cosmetic products can prevent this natural decline of skin elasticity – we can only help to preserve what we have. It is mostly the damage to the deeper layers that will determine how our skin looks as we get older, and this is largely self-inflicted because we over-expose ourselves to the sun.

Before we can discuss how to take care of skin we have to understand what it is and how it works.

What skin looks like

Seen from a distance, skin may look perfectly smooth. But what we actually see is dependent

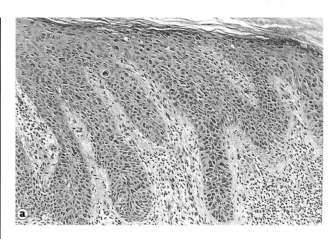

The skin has a complex structure below its surface, seen here under the microscope.

on several factors, including the state of the very top layer, the type and amount of pigment in the layers beneath and the state of the tissues and the blood vessels in the deeper layers.

As we get nearer it becomes obvious that the skin is not absolutely smooth and perfect.

If we look even more closely we will see that the surface is marked by a network of tiny furrows of variable sizes which divide the surface into rough rectangles. These change shape during movements of the skin. In some areas, such as the hands, movement would not be possible without the flexibility afforded by these furrows.

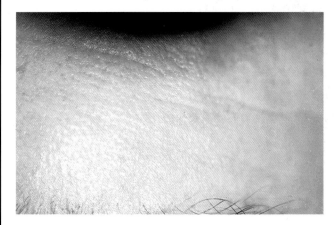

Looking closely at older skin reveals fine lines and pores.

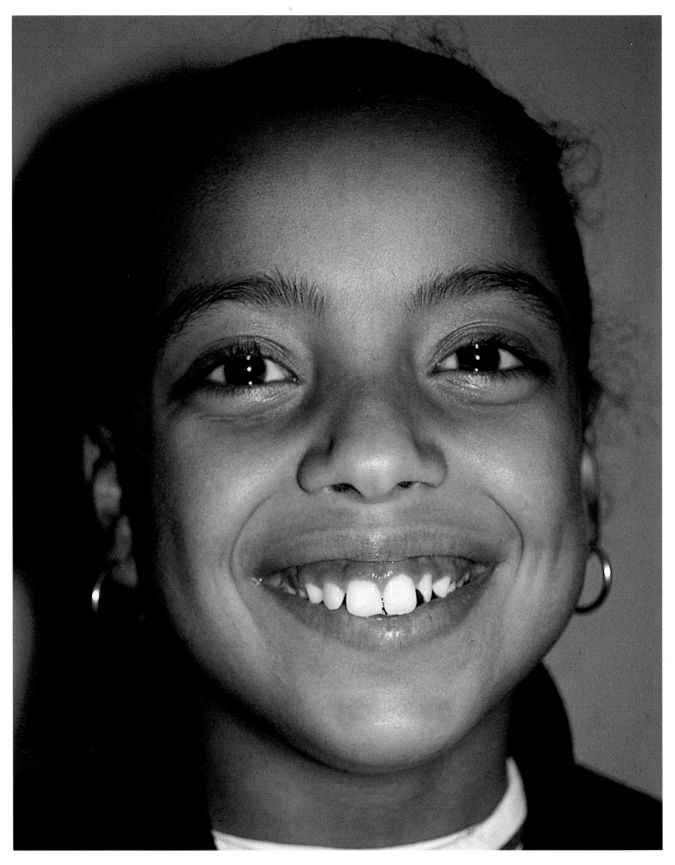

First impressions may depend on the condition of the skin of the face. In youth light is reflected from a healthy, undamaged skin that is functioning perfectly.

SKIN FACTS

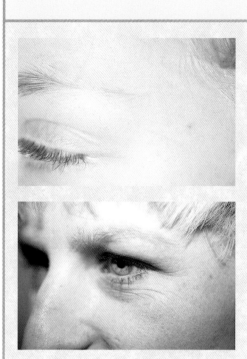

◄ The delicate skin around the eyes undergoes some marked changes over the years: this shows the eyes of an eight-year-old...

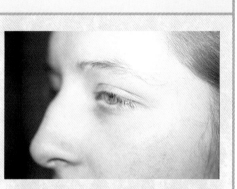

...but at the age of 20 early ▶ signs of damage are visible...

◄ ...and by 34 fine lines and wrinkles are developing...

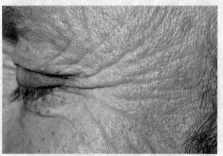

...which have deepened into ▶ crows' feet by the age of 60. These are mainly due to exposure to ultraviolet light; daily protection with products containing UV sunscreens may help to reduce them.

- The skin covering the body of a newborn baby has an area of about 2500 cm². By the time the baby has grown up it may have to cover 18 000 cm² (1.8 square metres – about the size of a shower curtain). If the baby grows up to be very tall or very fat, it can be considerably more.

- The skin of an average woman weighs about 3 kg, and that of an average man perhaps 5 kg.

- The thickness of the skin varies, depending on its site on the body. It is thinnest on the eyelids and thickest on the palms of the hands and the soles of the feet.

Over most of the body the skin carries hairs, but in most people these are not very noticeable except on the head, eyebrows, eyelids, face, armpits and groin. In some dark-haired people the hairs on the forearms and legs (and, in men, the chest) may be visible. Shaving leg hair is common in some cultures.

There are sweat glands all over the skin, opening at tiny pores on the surface; in certain areas, such as the armpit, they are particularly prominent.

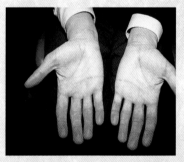

Thick skin on the palms of the hands can withstand considerable wear and tear...

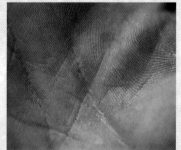

...and may develop callouses (patches of hard, horny skin) to protect the structures beneath.

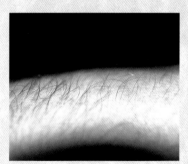

'Terminal' hairs grow on the scalp and eyebrows. After puberty they also grow in areas that are sensitive to sex hormones.

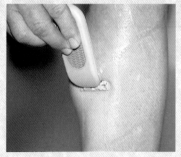

Smooth-skinned legs are seen as attractive in some but not all cultures. Shaving does not make hairs grow more strongly: it just feels that way.

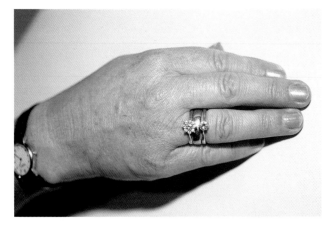

The skin over the fingers owes much of its flexibility to the arrangement of deeper tissues overlaying the joints...

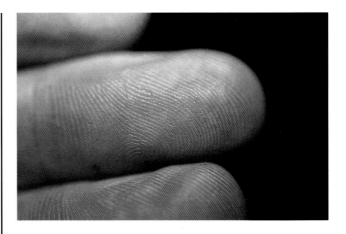

Everyone carries complex and unique skin patterns on their fingertips.

On the face there may be many deeper wrinkles, particularly around the eyes. These become more marked with age and are significantly deepened by sun exposure and smoking.

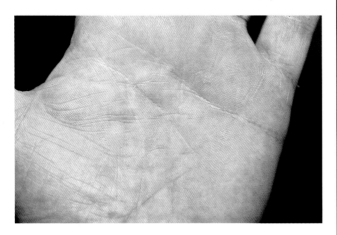

...while the folds in the thick skin of the palms allow the hands to open and close freely.

Skin furrows are most obvious over the joints, where they correspond with folds in the deeper layers of the skin caused by joint movements. The lines on the back of the hand are quite faint, and cross each other at various angles.

There are also skin lines that are normally invisible but become apparent in certain rare pigmentation disorders (see page 29). The lines on the palms of the hand and the fingers (and on the soles of the feet) are fine but very distinct, making a series of parallel curves and forming patterns which are unique to each individual ('fingerprints'). These are caused by the peculiar arrangement of the deeper parts of the skin. The pores of the sweat glands open on the ridges of these patterns.

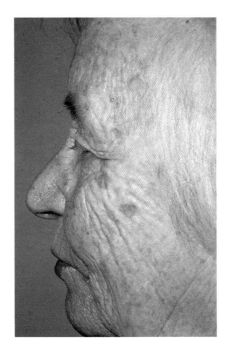

Damage due to sunlight changes the age at which skin patterns become seriously altered...

In skin heavily affected by the sun patterns emerge, both coarse and fine.

When we look at skin under a microscope it looks almost like a moon landscape, with hairs growing out of it. The patterns are more obvious and flakes of dead skin can be seen.

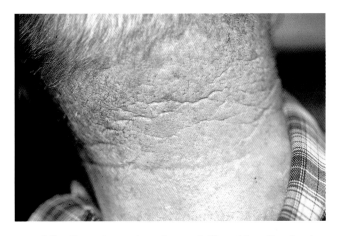

...and fine lines change into deep wrinkles: this – the classic 'red neck' – is the effect of a lifetime in the sun.

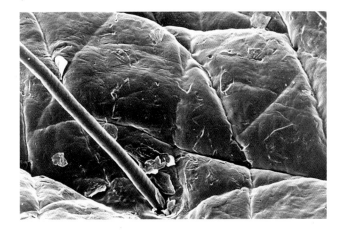

Seen with an electron microscope, skin looks almost like a lunar landscape; a growing hair can be seen among the 'rocks', which are dry, dead skin cells called 'squames'.

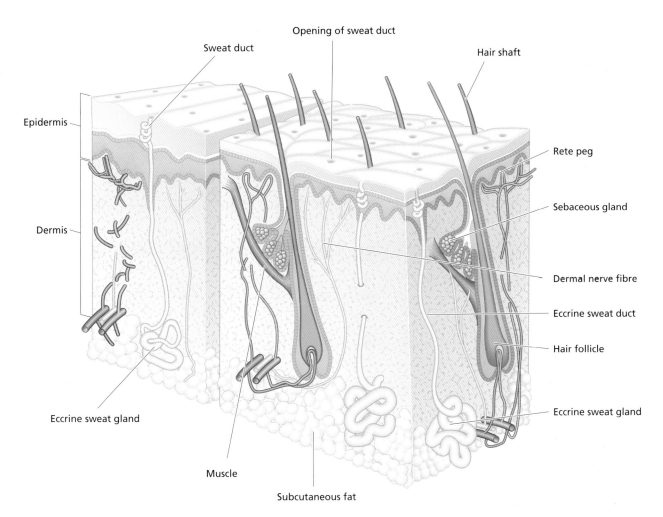

The three-dimensional structure of the skin, shown diagrammatically: (left) the thick hairless skin of the palm of the hand, (right) the thin hairy skin of the forearm.

The layers of the skin

The skin is made up of three distinct layers.

The top layer is called the **epidermis**. (The word *epidermis*, and the name of the other main skin layer, the *dermis*, both come from the name used by the ancient Greeks for the skin, *derma*. From this we also get the word *dermatologist*, meaning a doctor who specialises in skin problems.)

The epidermis is translucent. That is, it allows light to pass partially through it, rather as frosted glass does. The epidermis does not contain any blood vessels but gets its oxygen and nutrients from the deeper layers of the skin.

At the bottom of the epidermis is a very thin membrane, called the **basement membrane**, which attaches the epidermis firmly, though not rigidly, to the layer below.

The second layer lies deeper and is called the **dermis**. It contains blood vessels, nerves, hair roots and sweat glands.

Below the dermis lies a layer of fat, the **subcutaneous fat**. The depth of this layer differs from one person to another. It contains larger blood vessels and nerves, and is made up of clumps of fat-filled cells called **adipose cells**.

The subcutaneous fat lies on the muscles and bones, to which the whole skin structure is attached by connective tissues. The attachment is quite loose, so the skin can move fairly freely. If the subcutaneous tissues fill up with too much fat the areas of attachment become more obvious and the skin cannot move as easily – this is what gives rise to the notorious **cellulite** (see pages 32 and 34).

The junction between the epidermis and the dermis is not straight but undulates like rolling hills – more markedly so in some areas of the body than others. A series of finger-like structures called **rete pegs** project up from the dermis, and similar structures project down from the epidermis. These projections increase the area of contact between the layers of skin, and help to prevent the epidermis from being sheared off. They are not present in the skins of unborn babies but rapidly develop after birth, and are very noticeable in a young person's skin when it is examined under the microscope. As skin ages they get smaller and flatter.

Networks of tiny blood vessels run through the rete pegs, bringing food, vitamins and oxygen to the epidermis. In pale people these vessels can be seen through the epidermis, particularly if the veins widen (so-called 'broken veins'). If the blood carries plenty of oxygen it will be pink and the skin will tend to have a rosy colour. If the blood is running sluggishly and has lost most of its oxygen the skin will look bluer. These blood vessels respond to temperature changes. They open up in hot weather, bringing lots of red blood cells – and hence a pink flush – to the skin, and close down in the cold; this is why cold skin often looks blue.

In most areas of the body the epidermis is only 35–50 micrometres thick. (A **micrometre** is one-millionth of a metre – one-thousandth of a millimetre.) On the palms and the soles it is usually much thicker, up to several millimetres. In the area around the eye it is only about 20 micrometres thick. This helps to explain why

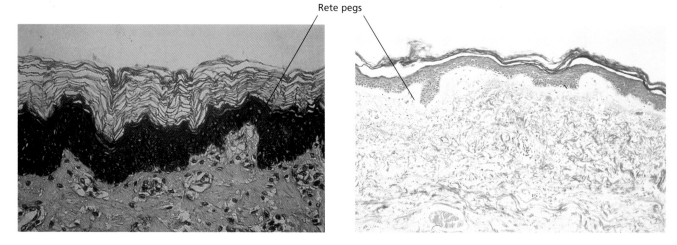

Rete pegs

(Left) One of the rete pegs that project into the dermis; (right) as we get older the rete pegs get smaller and flatter – this means the epidermis is more easily sloughed off in old age.

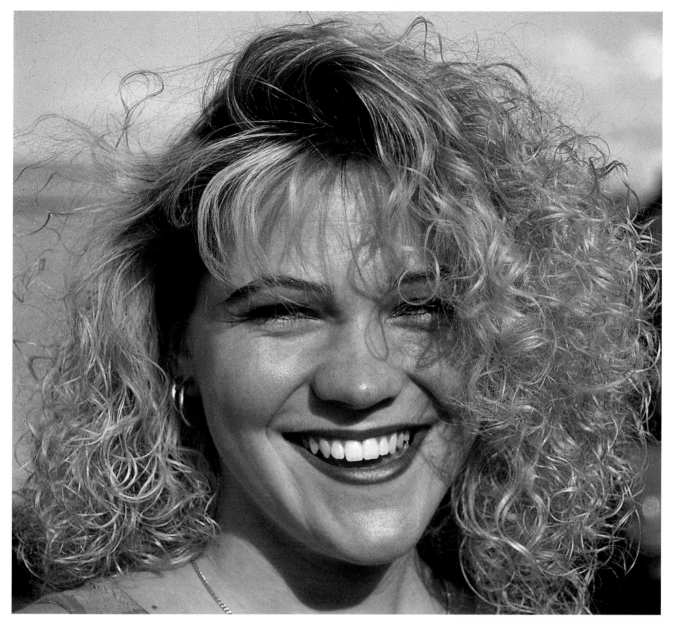

In young healthy skin a rise in external temperature, or hot food, brings a flow of blood to the many blood vessels in the cheeks.

the skin around the eye is so very sensitive: irritating substances have to penetrate the epidermis before they can affect the underlying skin, so the thinner the epidermis the less resistant to irritants it will tend to be.

The epidermis around the eye is not only very thin; it also contains many blood vessels. 'Circles' or dark shadows under the eyes are possibly due to slow blood flow and the resulting build-up of lymph. This may also account for the puffy 'morning after' look.

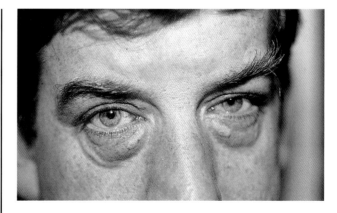

Heavy bags under the eyes; in this man they are accentuated by visible fat deposits.

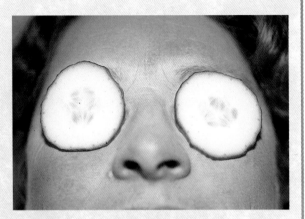
The epidermis

All the cells in the epidermis originate ultimately from a single layer of **basal cells**, called the **basal layer**, which sits on the basement membrane. The 'daughter cells' produced by this basal layer gradually move upwards, lose their central nucleus, and start to produce skin proteins called **keratins** (hair is made up of a similar, but harder, material) and fats called **lipids**. They are now known as **keratinocytes**. As they move upwards through the skin thickness their form slowly changes. The altered cells form distinct layers, which naturally blend into each other.

As the daughter cells move upwards their shape flattens, and they become joined by spiny

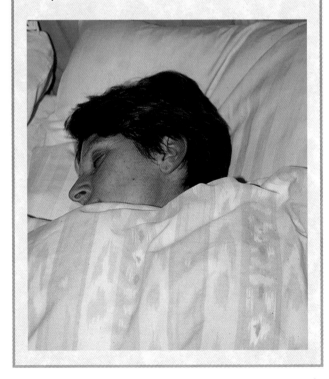
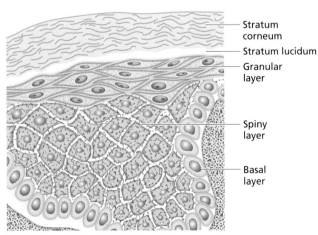

Stratum corneum
Stratum lucidum
Granular layer
Spiny layer
Basal layer

The layers of the epidermis

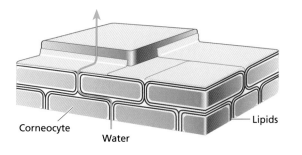

A model of the 'bricks and mortar' arrangement of the cells of the stratum corneum. The flattened cells (corneocytes) are held together by attachments called desmosomes. The lipids (natural fats) between them help to conserve moisture since water cannot pass through them easily.

Corneocyte

Water

Lipids

processes to make another recognisable layer, known as the **spiny layer**. These cells make special fats called **sphingolipids**. When the cells reach the stratum corneum these lipids will play an important part in the retention of moisture in the skin.

As the cells migrate further upwards they develop characteristic granules; they now form part of the **granular layer**. In the upper cells of this layer these granules discharge and fill up the spaces between the cells with lipids,

ultimately creating an appearance of a wall of bricks (cells) and mortar (lipids).

As the cells rise into the top layer of the epidermis – the **stratum corneum**, sometimes called the **horny layer** or the **cornified layer** – they take the form of flattened discs, tightly packed together. These flattened cells, now called **corneocytes**, are effectively dead. The number of layers of cells in the stratum corneum depends on the site on the body; on the sole of the foot the stratum corneum is at its thickest, and is there made up of hundreds of layers of densely packed cells.

The stratum corneum acts as an outer 'covering' to the skin, able to resist scrapes and scratches on the outside and helping to keep water on the inside. In this respect it is rather like the bark of a tree.

Throughout a person's life, from birth to death, the cells of this layer are continually being worn away and replaced from below with new cells. The wearing process is called **desquamation**, and the flattened scales of

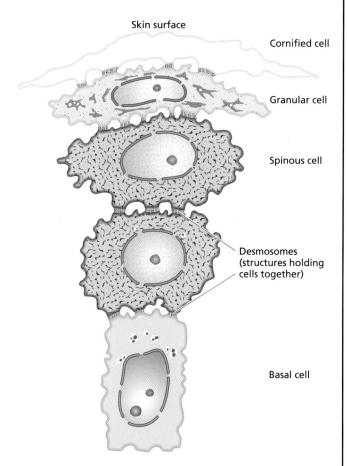

Skin surface

Cornified cell

Granular cell

Spinous cell

Desmosomes (structures holding cells together)

Basal cell

The different forms of the cells of the epidermis: as the cells move upwards they gradually change shape.

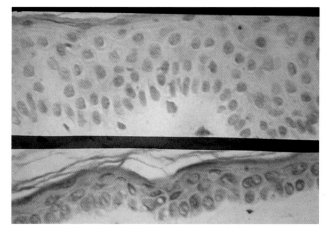

Sections of the epidermis, compared: (top) aged 18, (bottom) aged 80. The reasons why the epidermis changes throughout life are discussed in Chapter 4, 'Skin and ageing'.

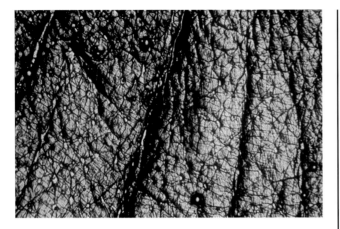

The stratum corneum acts as an outer 'hide' that can resist injury and help to conserve water in the skin.

dead skin are called **squames** (see page 9). Each squame is only about a micrometre thick but some 35 micrometres across. Desquamation tends to slow down as we grow older. In any particular part of the body, however, the results of the processes of cell loss and replacement are that the skin tends to remain the same overall thickness.

In normal skin, it takes about 30 days for a cell produced by the basal layer to move through the epidermis to the surface. The rate of movement is partly controlled by the rate at which the outer layer is being lost. When stratum corneum cells are being lost quickly – perhaps after sunburn – they are replaced more quickly from below. In skin that has been injured (grazed, for instance) the process speeds up dramatically. Artificially removing the outer layers by the cosmetic process of peeling (**exfoliation**) also tends to speed up replacement.

The stratum corneum is a very important layer from the point of view of understanding skin, skin problems, skin care and the beneficial effects of cosmetics such as moisturisers. It is the part of the skin that forms the junction of the body with the outside world, and it is directly affected by the outside environment, by harsh soaps, by skin care products and by the sun.

It plays a key role in helping to contain moisture within the rest of the skin, and in regulating the natural moisture flow out from the deeper layers to be lost eventually by evaporation from the skin surface. This flow is known as **transepidermal water loss** (TEWL), and it is important to understand the factors that influence it. Without adequate retained moisture skin can become dry and unhealthy.

Under normal conditions up to 15% of the stratum corneum consists of water. This water is vital to enable the stratum corneum itself to work. The natural functions of the skin do not work as well when the stratum corneum contains less than 10% of water, and it becomes dry.

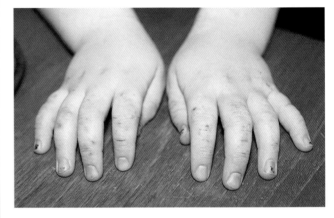

Unusually dry skin on the hands of a young child, requiring regular and generous moisturising.

In the epidermis the spaces between the cells are packed with fats, or **lipids**, made by the body. One very important group of these lipids is the **ceramides**, which are also ingredients of some skin care products.

The lipids of the epidermis play a vital role in healthy normal skin, as they help the stratum

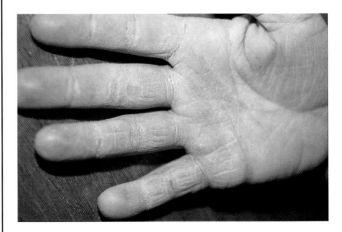

Removal of lipids leads the stratum corneum to break down.

corneum to regulate natural water loss. If they are removed by harsh soaps or detergents, or by damage such as a burn, the skin loses some or all of its ability to retain water, becomes dry and will start to break down.

The epidermis also contains natural **enzymes**, which are important for getting rid of old skin cells. Enzymes need moisture in which to work, so dryness (desiccation) of the stratum corneum worsens dry and unhealthy looking skin.

The pictures (below) of skin from the palm of the hand illustrate how the condition of the stratum corneum can vary. One is dry and the stratum corneum is not well hydrated: the other has been moisturised and the layer is now healthy. The same can be true of the skin of the face.

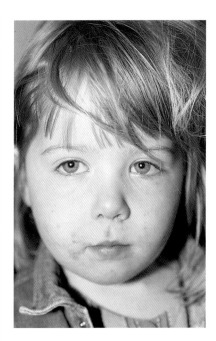

Even very young children may have dry skin.

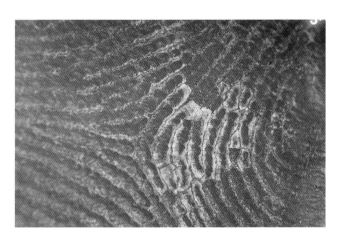

Parched, dry skin on the hands...

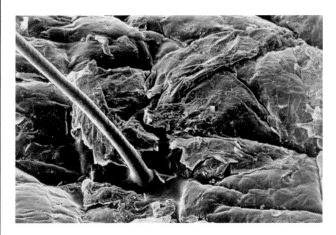

Seen still more closely, facial skin can be equally dry (as seen here)...

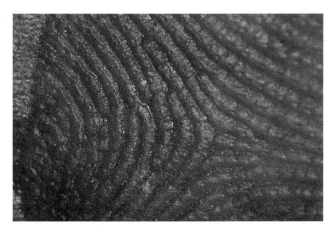

...can be improved by treating with moisturiser.

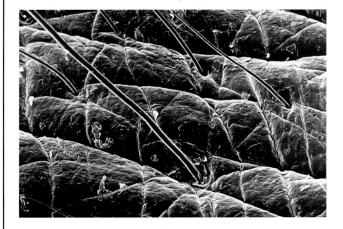

...but again its surface can be smoothed out with a good moisturiser.

Skin colour

The keratinocytes are not the only cells in the epidermis.

Among the most important of these cells are the **melanocytes**, which are found in the basal layer of the epidermis. These manufacture a special pigment called **melanin**, which helps to determine the colour of the skin and hair. The

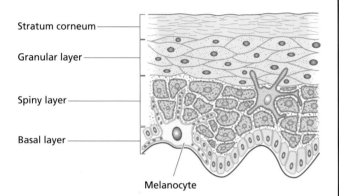

The melanocytes of the epidermis are crucial in determining skin colour.

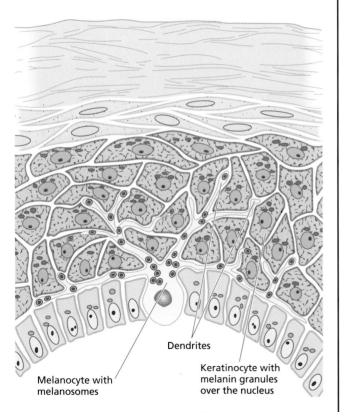

The distribution of melanin in the epidermis.

pigment is made on tiny structures called **melanosomes**, which aggregate as granules and are delivered in small 'packages' to each basal cell by slender filaments called **dendrites**. One melanocyte supplies about 36 keratinocytes with melanin granules. These tiny packages of pigment sit over the nucleus – the vital centre of the cell – in every cell in the epidermis, and protect it from the harmful rays of the sun.

Over-exposure to strong sunlight may damage the basal cell nuclei so badly that they produce abnormal 'daughter cells' that eventually turn into cancer cells. A similar problem is met with by some people who have no pigment in their skin or hair (**albinos**), and therefore have no natural protection against the sun. Albino people must be especially careful to protect their skin.

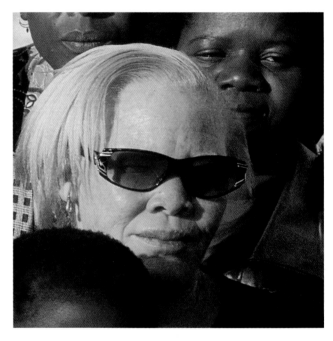

This albino lady's African descent is visible in her features, but she has almost no pigment in her skin.

Melanin

There are two forms of the pigment melanin: **eumelanin** granules, which tend to be round and smooth and produce black and brown skin colours, and **phaeomelanin** granules, which are more irregular in shape and which are more prominent in lighter skins, particularly in association with red hair and freckles.

These two forms of melanin are often both present together, and occur in varying proportions.

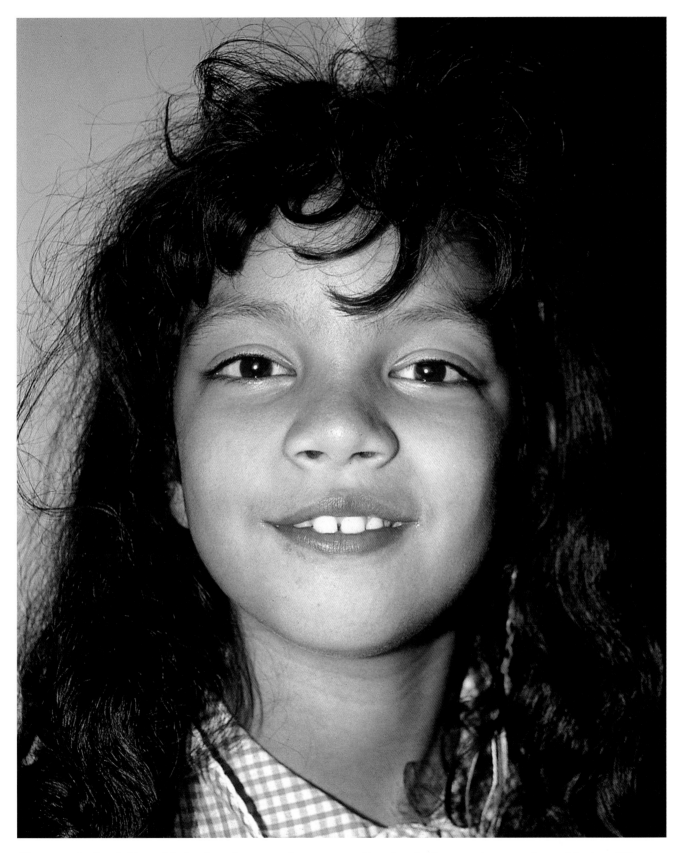

The many shades of skin and hair colour that we see in any group of people arise from varying proportions of the two different melanin pigments. A high proportion of eumelanin leads to darker skin and (particularly) hair colour; people with lighter skin and hair have less eumelanin and more phaeomelanin.

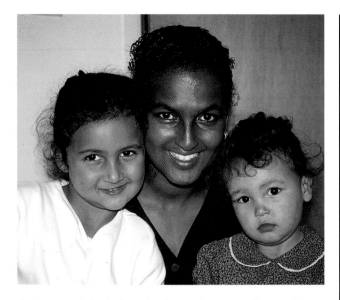

(Above and below) Melanins in varying proportions and concentrations.

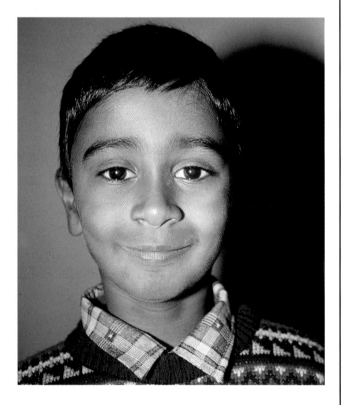

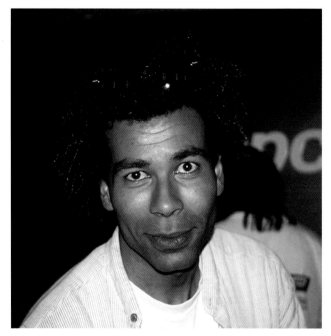

Although of Danish nationality, this man is of mixed Caucasian and African descent. His skin colour, as well as other characteristics, result from his genetic make-up.

Differences in skin colour
Eumelanin is the commoner and more dominant pigment of the two, particularly in hair. Most of the world's people have black hair, but skins that range from very fair to black.

Skin colour and hair colour tend to go together and may reflect our ancestors' adaptation to their environment. Scientists believe that the earliest humans originated hundreds of thousands of years ago in an area now found in the African continent. The gradual evolution of the human race continued along different lines, until there were essentially three different ancestral racial groups:

- Mongoloid – Oriental peoples
- Negroid – people of direct African descent.
- Caucasian – including the people of north-western Europe and also very dark-skinned Indians

Melanin production in skin varies in the three racial groups. 'Black' skins do not contain any more *melanocytes* than white ones do. But there are differences in the *melanin* granules in the differently coloured skins. In black skins the granules are larger, whereas in white skins they are less obvious.

- In Oriental people the melanosomes are relatively large in size, and are distributed within the skin cells as a mixture of single and complex forms.
- In Negroid skin the melanosomes are even larger; they are heavily pigmented and scattered singly throughout the keratinocytes.
- In white Caucasian skin the melanosomes are smaller and have less melanin; they are distributed as clumps in keratinocytes.

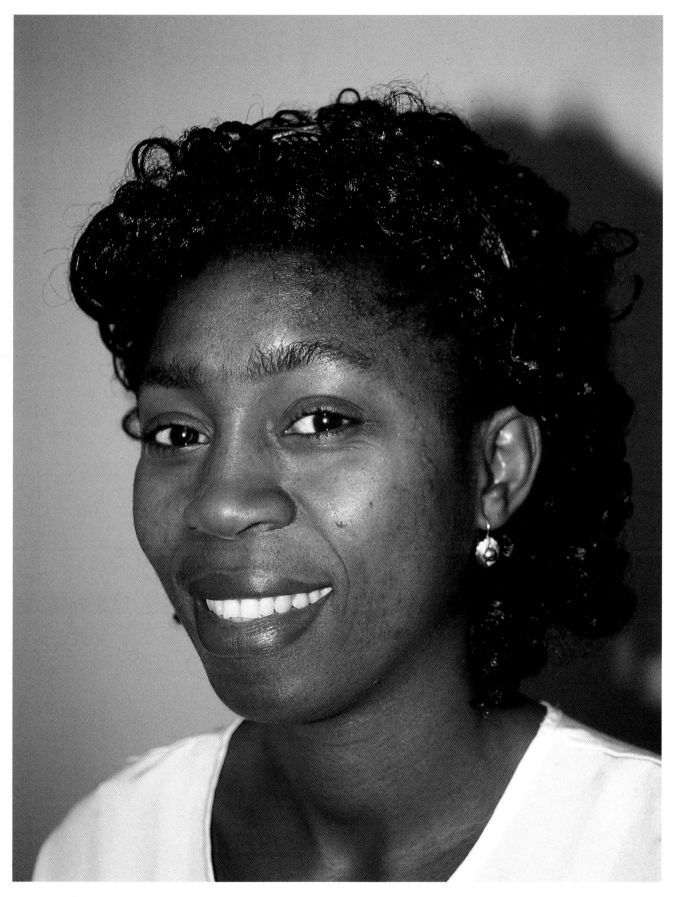

This Nigerian lady's skin contains heavy concentrations of eumelanin right through the epidermis.

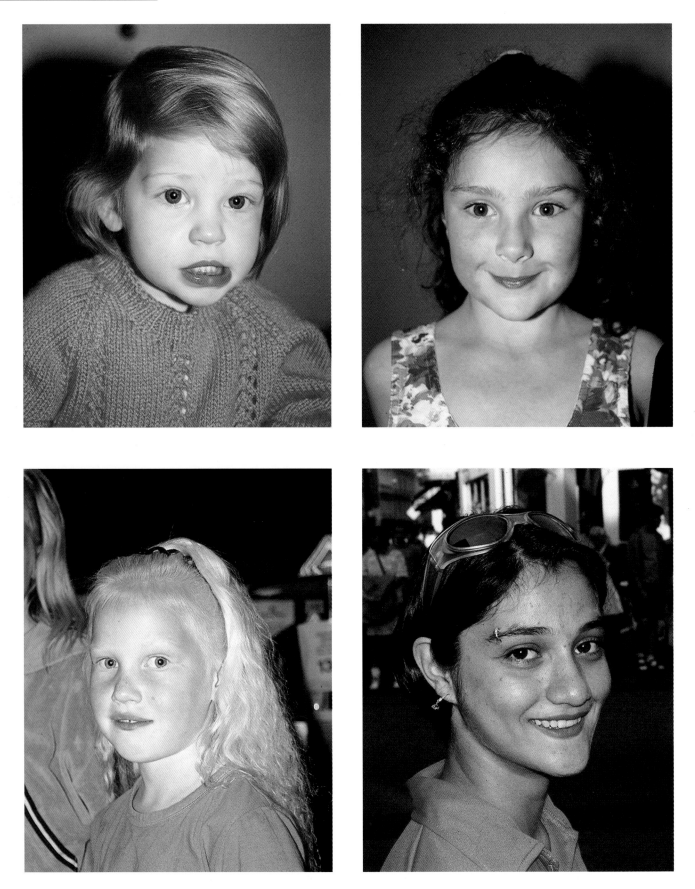

In Caucasian skins the proportions of the two main melanin pigments, eumelanin and phaeomelanin, vary over a huge range.

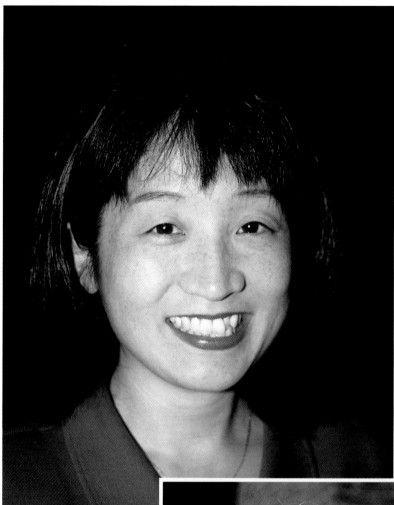

This Japanese woman has pale skin despite her hair colour.

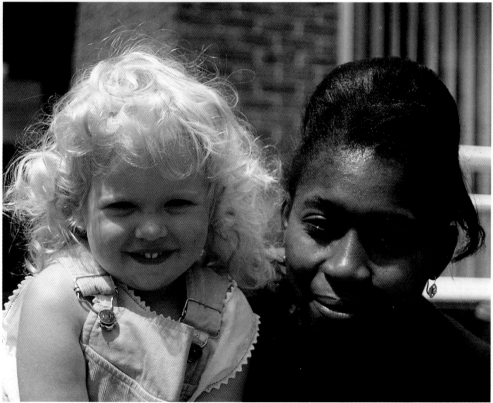

Our skin colour is the result of our genetic inheritance.

In equatorial regions of Africa, Latin America and India, where there is a high degree of sun exposure, many of the indigenous people have highly pigmented and thick skins that protect them from the harmful rays of the sun – very dark skin offers about 30 times more protection against the sun than pale skin does.

There is not, however, a definite relationship between skin pigmentation and the degree of exposure to sunlight. There are people with unexpected skin colours for the area in which they live. For example, the Tasmanian Australoids are dark-skinned although they live in a temperate latitude; also the pigmentation of American Indians, who are descendants of Mongol peoples, is similar across the whole continent of North America. These examples are probably the result of migrations forty or fifty thousand years ago. A few thousand years ago, unknown factors triggered a great migration of people from east to west. The native peoples of central and western Europe were pushed westwards. Among these were the original Celts (people with blue eyes and very pale skins easily burnt by the sun), who eventually populated parts of Scotland and Ireland; their descendants can still be identified in those countries.

Similarly, in the last few hundred years peoples with white skins have migrated to Australia and South Africa – areas of high sunshine to which their skins are not well adapted, and among them sun damage and skin cancer rates are high.

Some skin types appear to show specific and curious adaptations to their climate. Many Scandinavian people have pale skins and light hair in winter. In the short but sunny summer, many of them tan quite markedly and quickly while their hair bleaches to almost white.

In the last few centuries, increasing ease of travel and the creation of multinational countries such as the USA have led to a wide range of different shades of skin and hair types and colours among the world's population.

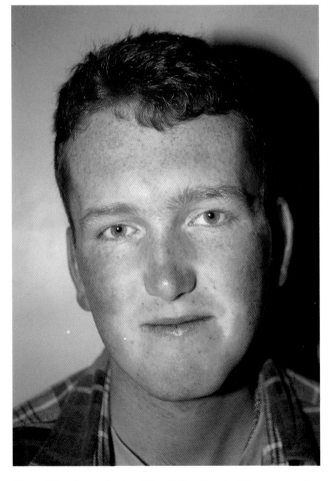
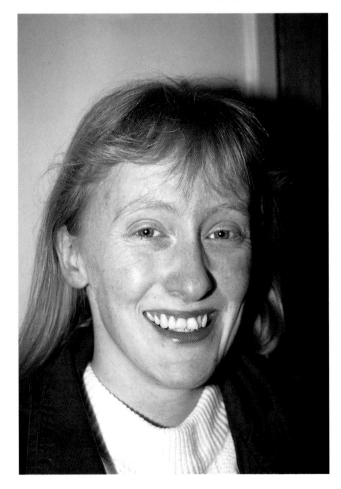

Two of the descendants of the Celts of central Europe: most are light- or red-haired, with skins that seldom tan but are easily sunburnt. This type of skin is prone to irritation.

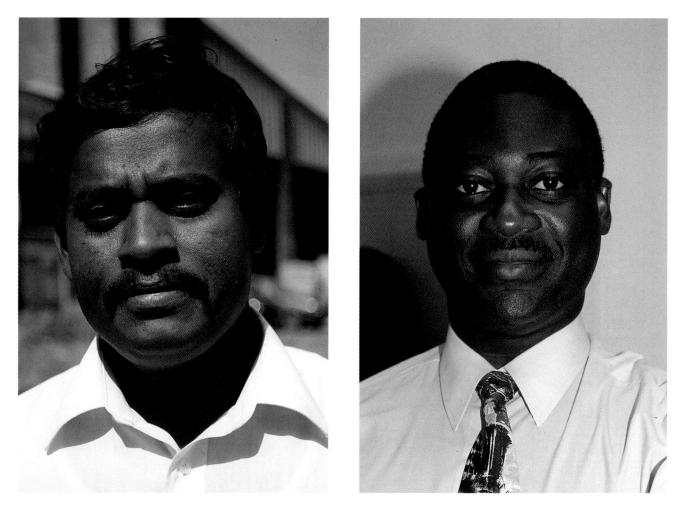

African and Indian peoples evolved heavily pigmented skins; but not all scientists are convinced that dark skin evolved only as an adaptation for sun protection. The bushmen of central Africa have dark skins, but live in tropical rainforest where there is little exposure to sunlight.

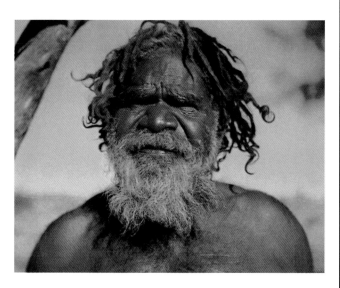

One of the dark-skinned race that has inhabited Australasia for thousands of years. They migrated there from Polynesia, but are related to African peoples.

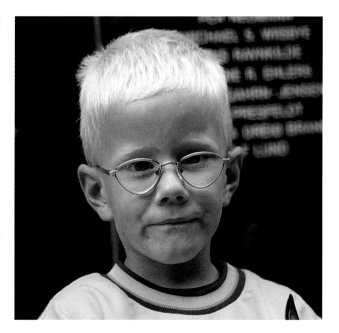

A child of the short Scandinavian summer, with a deep sun tan and nearly white hair.

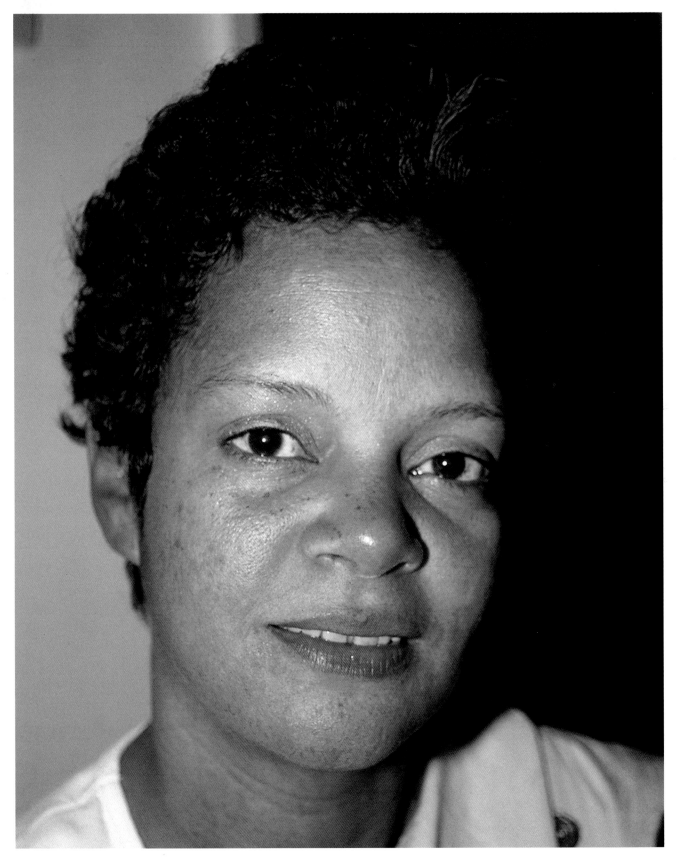

This lady's skin and features reflect the mixed African and European Colonial background of her birthplace. Such mixtures of characteristics are seen increasingly frequently all over the world.

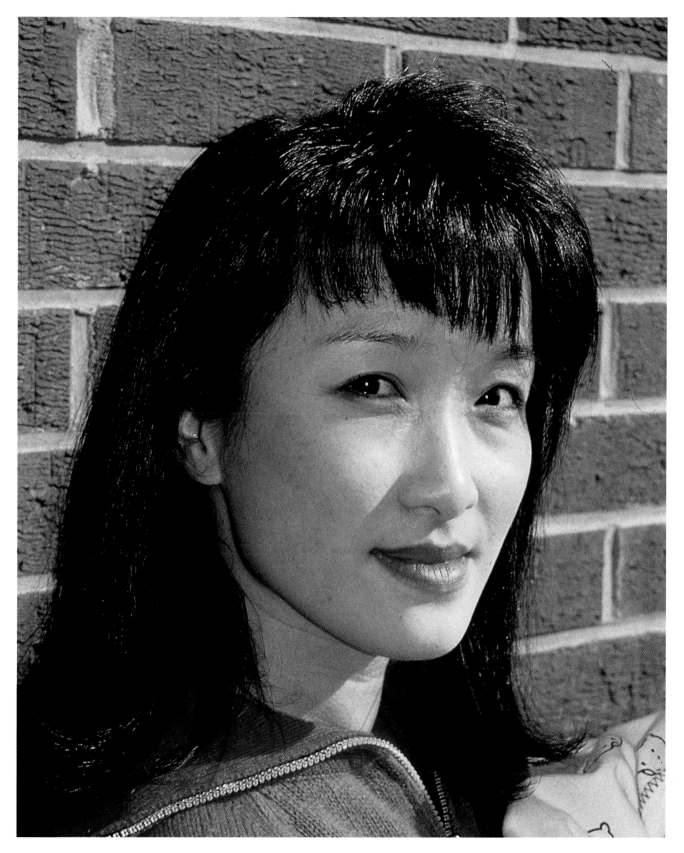

One quarter of the world's population inhabits the Chinese region. The 'yellow' colour of this lady's skin is probably due to a specific type of light absorption by the melanin in Mongoloid skin, which can vary from very light to dark, depending on the amount of pigment.

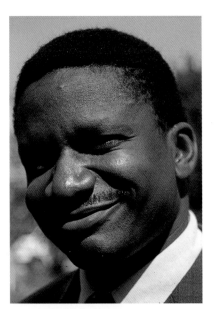

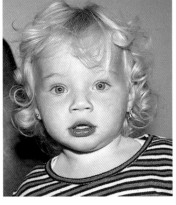

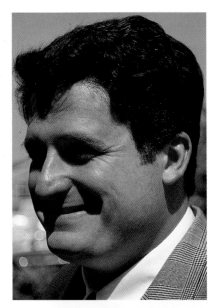

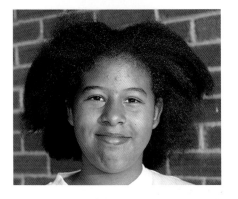

Skin types from all round the world: a tiny fraction of the enormous range.

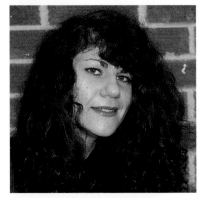

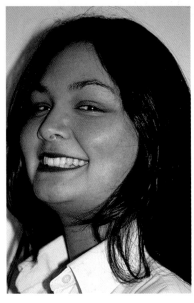

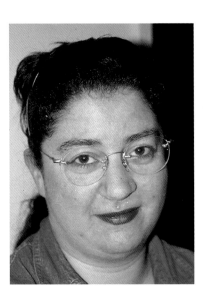

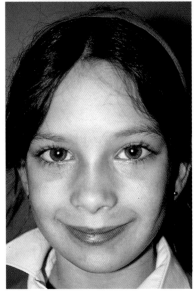

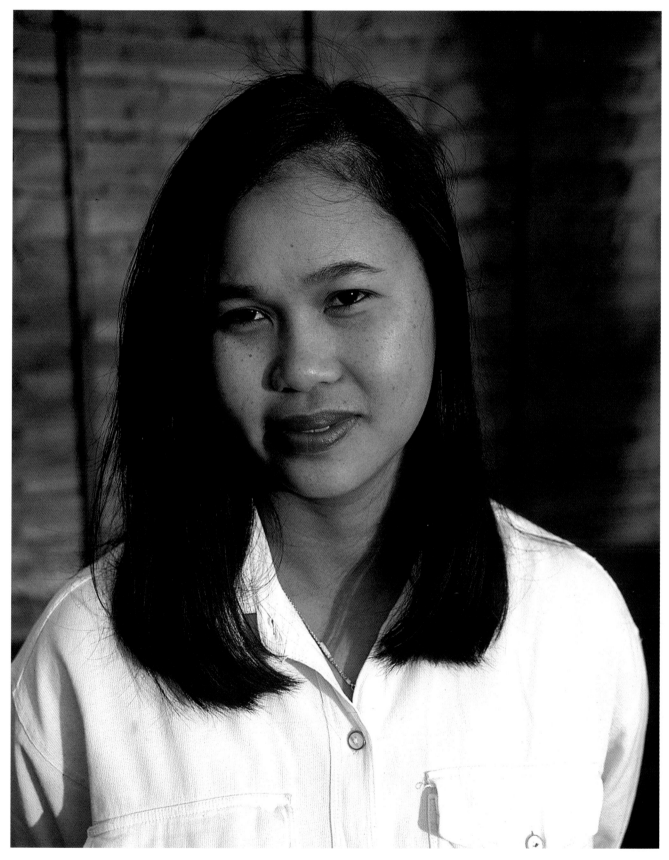

South-east Asia is one of the world's racial melting-pots, with a huge range of gene mixtures giving rise to many beautiful skin colorations.

Skin appearance and skin colour

When we look at skin many factors affect what we actually see, including the brightness and colour of the light, the state of the skin and the basic colour of the skin. These all combine to produce an effect that can alter dramatically.

In normal daylight, what we see is partly light reflected from the surface of the stratum corneum and partly light reflected back from the dermis through the translucent epidermis. If the stratum corneum contains adequate moisture and the dead cells (squames) have been removed, it is more translucent and reflects light more evenly, giving the skin a 'shine'.

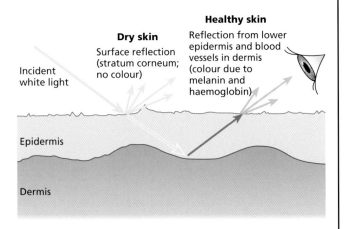

Model of the translucency of the skin.

If the skin is dry and covered in squames it scatters light instead of reflecting it evenly, and looks dull. (Much the same is true for hair.) If dry skin or hair is wetted with water, or better still with oil, it looks glossier because it reflects light better. This can be demonstrated very clearly on dry leather.

This also explains why moisturisers and exfoliators help skin to look healthier. They smooth down or remove the squames and help the epidermis to retain its moisture, so reflecting light better.

Changing this light reflection is a crucial part of what cosmetic products can do.

Very dark skins, with pigment throughout the epidermis, reflect less light from the dermis. But in skins with little or no pigment in the epidermis, the state of the tiny blood vessels in

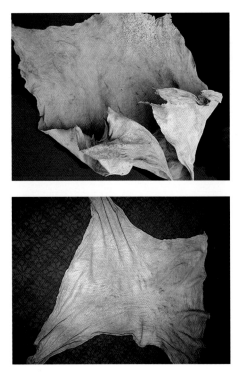

Our skin is not so very different from a 'leather': stiff and dull when dry, pliable and with a slight sheen when moist.

the dermis and the state of the dermis itself play a greater part in the 'complexion'.

What we see as the actual *colour*, as distinct from the *condition*, of our skin depends on light that is reflected by four different coloured components of the skin, which are found at different levels throughout the epidermis and the dermis. These reflections combine to give us our unique colour. They are:

- melanin in the epidermis
- red blood cells containing oxygen in the small blood vessels of the dermis
- red blood cells without oxygen in the same blood vessels
- orange-yellow chemicals called **carotenoids** in the stratum corneum and the subcutaneous fat layer; these are principally responsible for the yellow tones of skin colour, and are more abundant in men's skin than in women's.

Carotenoids are found in carrots.
Eating too many carrots can turn you orange!

Of these four factors, melanin is the most important in deciding skin colour. The

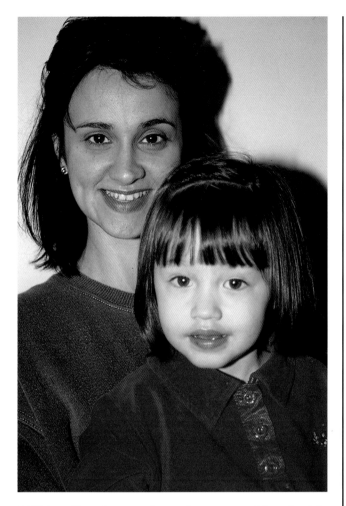

Differing skin colours are due to the presence of the coloured components of the skin in different proportions.

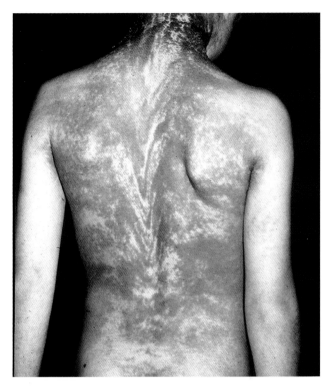

This abnormal pigmentation distribution follows lines of cells ('Blaschko's lines') that reflect developmental growth patterns.

out along the otherwise invisible lines on the skin called **Blaschko's lines**.

Vitiligo is a condition where there is patchy loss of pigment, usually over the hands and forearms but occasionally it is more extensive. It is possible to hide it by the skilful use of special water-resistant cosmetics.

contribution of blood to the complexion colour is most obvious in the cheeks, where capillaries are most numerous and closest to the surface.

Apparent skin colour can change if the combination of its coloured components changes. Changes like these are more obvious if very little melanin is present, since melanin can hide most of the other colours. This is why people with very pale skins – 'porcelain' skins – can look blue if they get cold: blood that moves sluggishly carries less oxygen, and so looks bluish rather than having the bright red colour that is given by full oxygenation.

Pigmentation disorders
There are some rare congenital pigmentary disorders of skin. In one, the pigment is spread

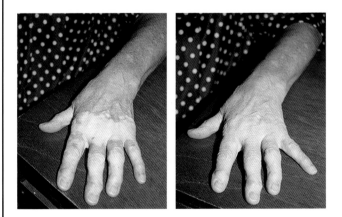

(Left) Vitiligo, a condition producing areas of unpigmented skin; (right) successful camouflage using special cosmetic products.

The dermis

Beneath the epidermis lies a much thicker skin layer, the dermis. The dermis can be as much as 3000 micrometres thick.

The dermis is composed largely of the protein **collagen**. Most of the collagen is organised in bundles running horizontally through the dermis, which are buried in a jelly-like material called the **ground substance**. Collagen accounts for up to 75% of the weight of the dermis, and is responsible for the resilience and elasticity of the skin.

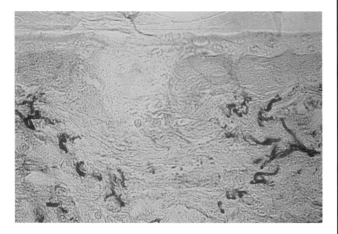

The ground substance of the dermis, seen under the microscope; it is an almost unstructured colloidal gel.

The collagen bundles are held together by **elastic fibres** running through the dermis. These are made of a protein called **elastin**, and make up less than 5% of the weight of the dermis. Despite their name, they are not involved in the natural elasticity of the skin.

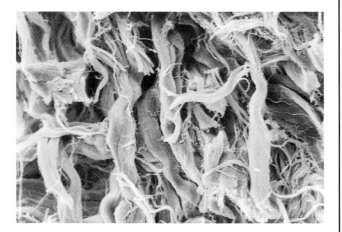

Massed collagen and elastin fibres in the dermis.

Both collagen and elastin fibres are made by cells called **fibroblasts**, which are scattered through the dermis.

Special substances in the ground substance, called **glycoproteins**, can hold large amounts of water, and are responsible for maintaining a mass of water in the dermis.

Hyaluronic acid is another important substance that forms part of the tissue that surrounds the collagen and elastin fibres. It has the ability to attract and bind hundreds of times its weight in water. In this way it acts as a natural moisturising ingredient responsible for the skin's plumpness and moisture reserve. As we get older the amount of hyaluronic acid produced in the skin naturally gets less. This is one reason why ageing skin becomes less resilient and supple (pliable). Recently

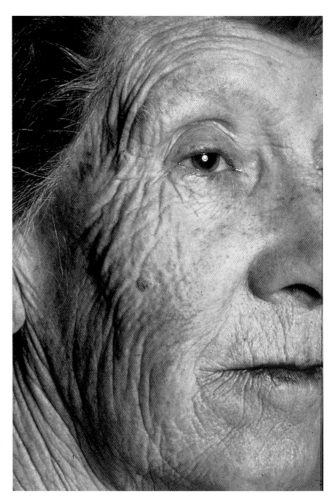

As skin gets older, it loses some of its elasticity and ability to retain water. Collagen production declines as does subcutaneous fat, and the facial muscles start to atrophy.

hyaluronic acid has been experimentally injected into skin, in an attempt to reduce wrinkles.

Another reason for skin ageing is that collagen and elastin production declines as the years go by, particularly after the menopause, so that some of the skin's natural properties are lost. (See also Chapter 4, 'Skin and ageing'.)

Injuries to the dermis

The deeper part of the dermis contains fewer blood vessels than the upper layers do, and many thick collagen bundles. These bundles lie parallel to each other along recognisable lines which are important to understand in wound healing. If a cut is made across these lines the skin gapes, and when the cut is healed there is more scarring than with wounds made along the lines of the bundles. Surgeons follow these lines when making their incisions, to ensure the best possible healing, which is why everyone's appendix scars are practically identical.

If the skin is seriously over-stretched, whether by too much fat or by pregnancy, the deep collagen fibres may actually rupture. This results in deep scars, which are seen through the intact epidermis as 'stretch marks'. Taking high doses of steroids for too long may have a similar result, as the collagen withers away (**atrophies**) under the influence of these drugs.

In a graze only the epidermis is sheared off. New epidermal cells very rapidly cover over the area with unscarred skin. Interestingly, these new cells are provided by cells from the hair follicles. Where a wound has damaged both the epidermis and the dermis, both the basal cells in the epidermis and the fibroblasts in the dermis go into intense production to seal the gap.

In a very narrow wound repair is relatively simple. But in large wounds the resulting repair is never perfect. **Granulation tissue** forms: this is a mixture of tiny blood vessels and fibroblasts frantically making collagen. This tissue eventually forms the scar: the greater the area to be covered, the larger will be the scar.

Sometimes the skin cells go on working at the repair process for much longer than necessary, so that far too much scar tissue is formed. This

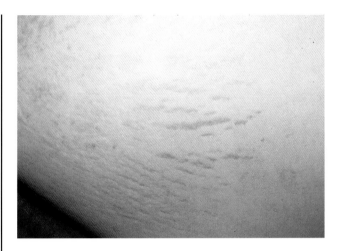

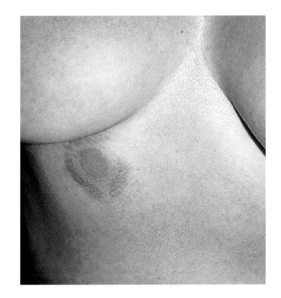

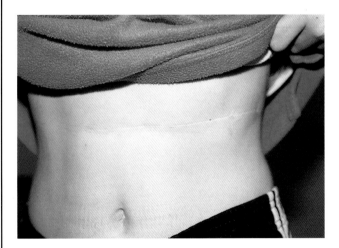

Different kinds of damage to the dermis: (top) stretch marks due to pregnancy; (middle) a burn – this will heal spontaneously; (bottom) a well-healed surgical scar.

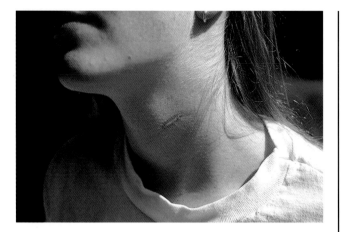

A keloid scar. Scars in older people tend to be cosmetically better.

produces a permanent raised scar called a **keloid**. Keloids are common with certain types of skin, particularly in young people and those from an African background. They can be injected with steroids by a doctor, which sometimes helps. Cutting them out is seldom effective, and usually makes them worse. Eventually they decrease in size.

Skin creases

In many regions of the body the skin is separated from the muscles by loose fatty tissue (of variable depth) and moves very easily. In other areas it is anchored to the bones. This is most obvious in the palms of the hands, where the skin is arranged so that it closely follows the movements of the fingers. Some of these creases form while a baby is still in the womb, or very soon after birth.

Folds and creases are also found on the face even in very young babies, as the skin accommodates the movements of the muscles of the face. In the face of a very fat person the subcutaneous layer of fat becomes thick and bloated, and reduces the appearance of these creases.

The subcutaneous fat layer

The subcutaneous fat layer cushions the dermis from underlying tissues such as muscle and bones.

As we have seen, this layer consists of cells containing fatty deposits, called adipose cells. The blood vessels and nerves it contains are larger than those in the dermis. It may also house the hair follicles when they are in the growing phase.

One of the functions of this fatty layer may be to act an insulation to conserve body heat. The human body stores fat as an energy reserve, in the same way that some animals store fat for winter when food supplies are likely to be short. Unfortunately the numbers of people with excess fat are increasing, thanks to their genetic predisposition together with habitually eating the now abundant sources of food. An excess of stored fat is seldom due to hormone problems, although as we get older fat deposition naturally increases as our metabolisms slow down. Getting normally heavier is therefore not necessarily due to us eating more food – just to eating.

Fat is stored *outside* the muscles. Although calorie reduction as part of an overall plan helps to make us slimmer, specific remedies to improve muscle tone in the tummy by exercise do not necessarily help to reduce the fat in that area. Distribution of fat in the body differs between men and women: in women it is stored mainly in the buttocks and thighs, and in men in the abdominal wall (the notorious 'beer belly').

The subcutaneous fat is organised into fat lobules, which are separated by collagen fibres. When these lobules become grossly distended and engorged by fat they adopt characteristic patterns (**cellulite**), in women particularly on the bottom and thighs where the skin is tethered down to the underlying muscles. These patterns tend to develop from the teens onwards.

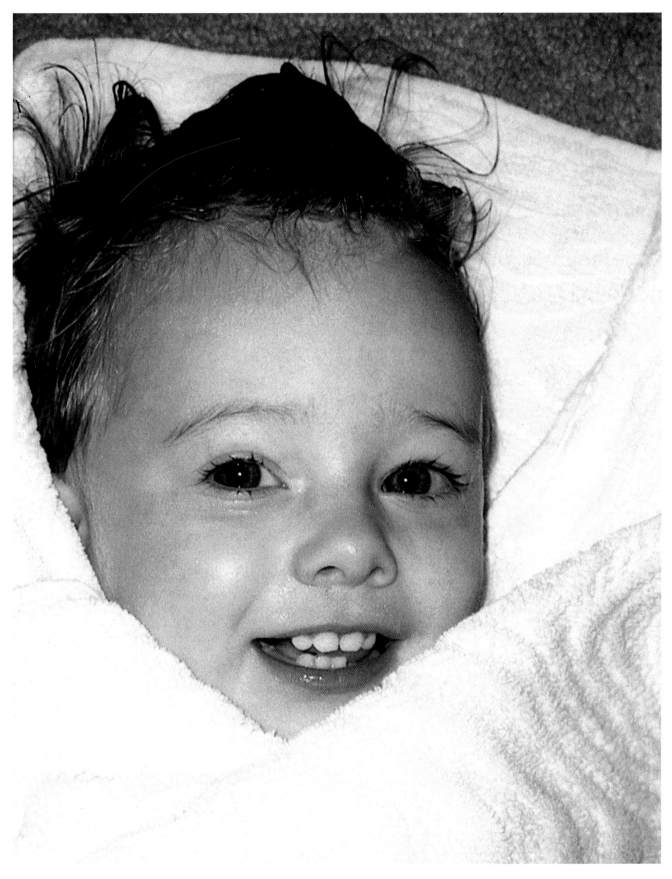

The skin of very young children is often plumped out with a generous layer of subcutaneous fat.

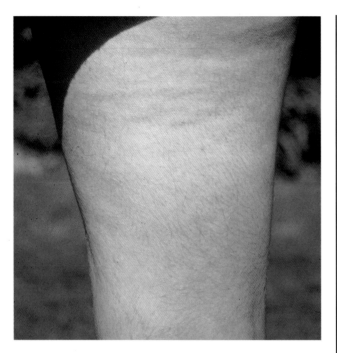

The dreaded cellulite is the result of genetically determined deposition of fat from the teens onwards.

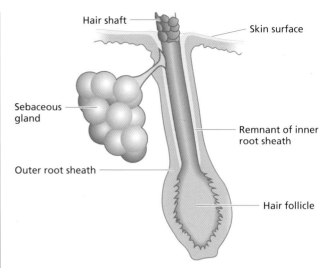

Sebaceous glands grow as part of the hair follicles. They produce sebum, which helps to protect the skin and lubricates the hair shaft.

There are no magic remedies for the selective elimination of this cellulite. It can only be reduced as part of an overall weight reduction program, together with cutting back on calorie intake and increasing exercise, although some fruit acid creams may help to make it temporarily less obvious.

Special skin structures

The skin contains certain important structures with special functions. The lips are specially developed as sense organs. The sweat glands help to regulate body temperature (see page 41). Most of the hairs on a human body have no real function and are a relic of when our ancestors needed warmer 'coats'.

The sebaceous glands

Sebaceous glands are part of the tiny structures – **hair follicles** – that generate hairs. These glands produce grease, or **sebum**, which is a mixture of waxes and fats. The glands empty through minute tubes called ducts. Sebaceous glands occur in the skin of every part of the body except on the palms and soles.

Sebum is secreted through the sebaceous duct into the hair follicle. It forms a mixture with the watery secretion of sweat, which covers the skin and spreads along the hair. The mixture of fat and water forms a natural oil-in-water emulsion (see pages 102–3) which may have a protecting action on the hair. It also kills some fungi that grow on the scalp.

Sebum is slightly acidic (pH between 4.2 and 5.6), which may be why people sometimes refer to the 'acid mantle' of the skin. This is a somewhat misleading expression in that it could wrongly suggest an impenetrable barrier. Skin is in fact permeable in both directions.

In both sexes the sebaceous glands are strongly influenced by male hormones, and are most sensitive to these at puberty, particularly on the face and trunk (the acne areas, see pages 56–7).

Sweat glands

Sweat glands are found in almost every part of the skin, forming tiny coiled tubes embedded in the dermis or subcutaneous fat. There are two types of sweat gland: **eccrine** glands and **apocrine** glands.

Eccrine glands produce sweat – a mixture of water and salts. Sweat plays an important part in regulating the temperature of the body by cooling it by evaporation of water from the skin

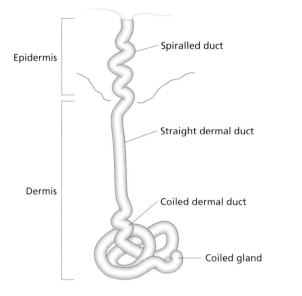

An eccrine sweat gland: most of the body's sweat production is the result of eccrine gland activity.

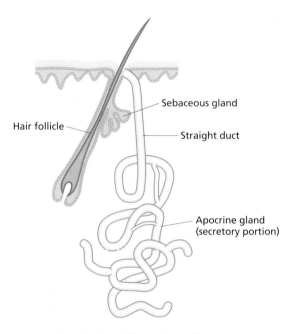

An apocrine gland, which produces little sweat but is responsible for the body's natural 'scent'.

(this is different from the transepidermal water loss through the stratum corneum). It also provides a useful natural method of removing waste products (toxins) from the body. The tiny ducts of the eccrine glands pass through the dermis and epidermis and empty directly on to the skin. They are found everywhere on the skin except on the lips and the glans penis.

Apocrine glands are formed from the same structure as the hair follicle and sebaceous glands. They produce a highly individual sexual scent, the production of which is dependent on the presence of sex hormones. The apocrine glands become very active with the onset of puberty. They are found particularly in the armpit and the genital area. The breasts are modified apocrine sweat glands.

Body odour is produced by micro-organisms ('germs') that grow in particularly moist areas of the skin, such as the armpit. They produce odour by digesting sebum, but they can only work efficiently if water is present. **Antiperspirants** can be used to reduce the amount of sweat produced in the armpit, where there are many sweat glands, and stop the germs growing rapidly. The role of antiperspirants is discussed in Chapter 5, 'Skin care'.

Hairs

Most of the skin is covered in fine hairs called **vellus hairs**, which are attached to tiny muscles in the dermis. When the air temperature falls, these muscles contract. When they do so the area in the skin to which they are attached is depressed and the skin around the hair 'stands up' – this produces 'goose bumps'. The process is of little or no value in helping us to keep warm.

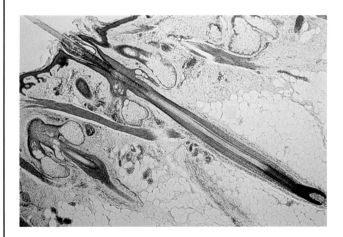

Section through a hair follicle buried deep in the subcutaneous fat of the scalp. When hair is about to fall out naturally this rises to the surface.

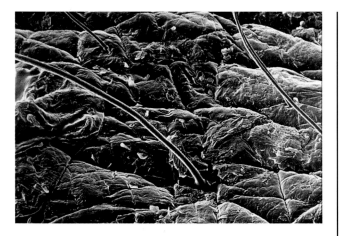

A hair growing from a follicle below the skin's surface.

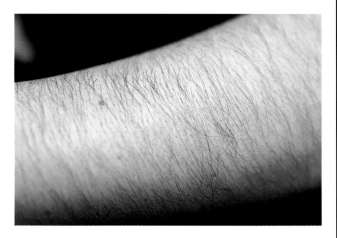

Fine vellus hairs grow all over the body except the palms and soles.

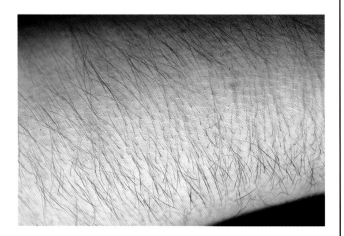

'Goose bumps' are due to depression of the skin as tiny muscles tighten and raise the hairs.

In babies and children longer, darker and thicker hairs, called **terminal hairs**, grow on the scalp, eyelids and eyebrows, though nowhere else. In the teens, however, the body starts to produce sex hormones. Both sexes produce some male hormones, and it is these that cause terminal hairs to develop in many other areas such as the beard area, chest, arms and legs. They do not replace the fine vellus hairs – they are still there as well.

Lips

The lips are prominent facial features. They can be divided into three different regions. There is skin on their outer surfaces and a thin smooth lining (**mucosa**) on the inner surfaces. Between these two tissues lies the **vermilion zone** (or red zone). It is this zone which people commonly call 'the lips'.

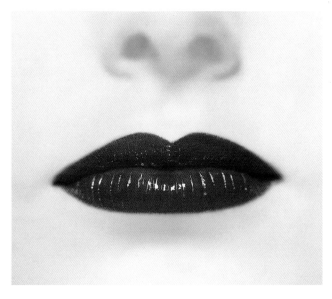

The vermilion zone of the lips can put out powerful signals; here the impression is hugely enhanced by a decorative cosmetic.

The vermilion zone forms the transitional zone between the mucosa of the mouth and facial skin. It shares some features with the facial skin that surrounds it, but also has some noticeable differences.

The skin of the lips, like skin elsewhere, has a dermis and an epidermis. The epidermis of the lips functions in a similar manner to the epidermis on other parts of the body: it provides a self-renewing barrier, protected from the outer world by a continually exfoliating stratum corneum. The characteristic red colour of the lips is unique to humans and comes from the blood vessels in the dermis. The many rete pegs (papillae) are long and narrow, and contain loops full of blood vessels. The closeness of these vessels to the surface, combined with a thin, almost transparent epidermis, gives rise to the red appearance of the lips. In cold weather when the blood vessels close down and the circulation becomes sluggish, the lips look blue.

The ridged appearance of the lips results from a highly folded dermis, which is not found in the skin of other parts of the body.

There are no hair follicles and sweat glands in the dermis of the lips – this is one of the most marked differences from other parts of the skin. The absence of these features within the lip dermis means that the lubricating effects of sebum are not present in the lips. As a result the lips can easily become dry and chapped. The stratum corneum of the lips is thinner than that of the rest of the skin, worsening this effect. The lips require constant re-hydration keep them healthy and to prevent drying, with the accompanying deterioration in appearance. As everyone has found, licking dry lips just makes the dryness worse. Only a product like a lip salve can help, because only this can ensure that water molecules accumulate effectively in the stratum corneum. Modern lipsticks can help to protect the lips.

Nails

The nails are flattened, elastic structures which are relics of claws. They consist largely of compressed keratin, and are in fact greatly

thickened areas of the epidermis. The keratin of the nails is derived from the **stratum lucidum** (meaning 'the clear layer'), which lies just below the stratum corneum (see page 12). The keratin of the nails can absorb large amounts of water, particularly during a warm soak. This is why nails are softer, and much easier to cut, after a bath.

On average, fingernails grow by half a millimetre or so a week; toenails grow a little more slowly. Growth is said to be quicker in the summer than in winter, and is most rapid in the longer digits.

The white flecks that sometimes appear in the nails are due to minute air bubbles in their structure.

Sex-related features of skin

There are subtle differences between the skins of men and women.

The stratum corneum tends to be thicker in men than in women. Moreover, in men the *total* skin thickness is about 25% greater than in women. The collagen content of skin is directly related to sex: male forearm skin, for example, contains more collagen than female skin at the same site at all ages.

There is also a difference in the composition of the sebum. Also, throughout their lives men produce more sebum than women do, and the lipid film on the surface of their skin is therefore more pronounced: as a result, desquamation in men is a slower process than it is in women.

There are also differences in sweat secretion between the sexes. Men have fewer sweat glands, both eccrine and apocrine.

Skin ageing has different features in men and women. These are discussed in Chapter 4 ('Skin and ageing').

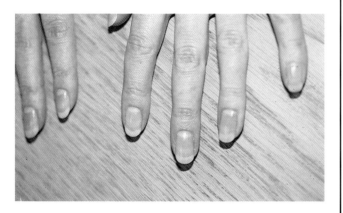

Well-cared-for nails enhance beautiful hands.

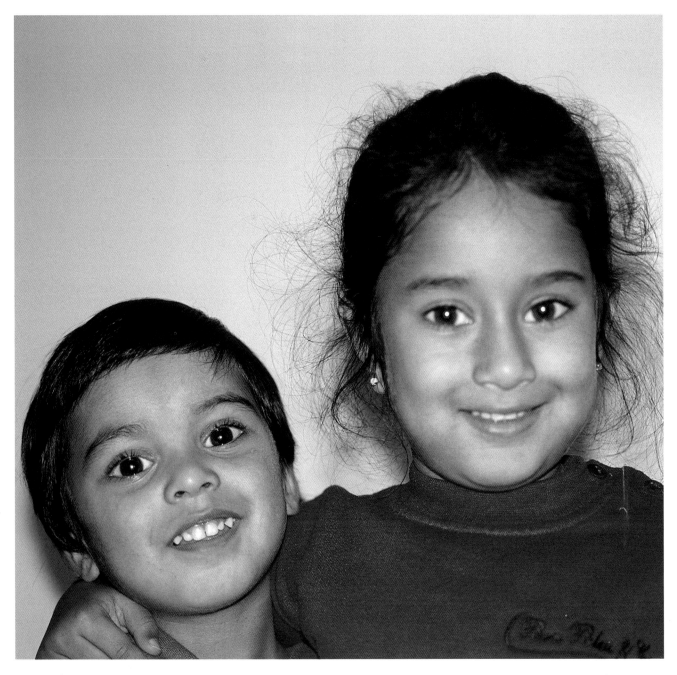

These beautiful Caucasian children (brother and sister) come from the original Indo-Aryan stock, whose descendants have populated a region stretching from western Europe to the Indian subcontinent.

2
Skin functions

Skin has many functions, and is far more than a mere decoration for the body. Some of these functions are so important that unless most of the skin is working efficiently, we will die.

This is the reason why second- or third-degree burns are so serious. When the skin is destroyed over a large area, there is no way of controlling the rate at which water is lost to the outside environment, or of regulating the temperature of the body or of controlling infection. Someone who has lost over half the skin this way is unlikely to survive.

Although we think of the skin as a single organ, the epidermis and dermis have to some extent separate functions. The function of water conservation is however dependent on both; the role of the stratum corneum in this field is absolutely vital, as it acts as a semipermeable barrier and allows us to survive in a hostile environment.

Functions of the epidermis

The epidermis has three principal functions:

- protecting the body from the environment, particularly the sun
- preventing excessive water loss from the body
- protecting the body from infection.

Protection from the environment

The sun produces enormous amounts of heat and light, some of which reaches the earth. Without this heat and light no life could ever have evolved.

Unfortunately the sun also produces less beneficial rays, which are completely invisible to us, called **ultraviolet radiation**. (Sun beds also expose their users to these rays.) Part of this radiation is reflected by the stratum corneum at the skin surface, part is absorbed by the melanin in the epidermal cells, and some is scattered within the skin. All three processes contribute to the vital function of protecting the nuclei of the cells in the epidermis and the collagen of the dermis.

This scattered radiation creates a lot of high-energy particles, which are called **free radicals**. Free radicals are very reactive, and attack the constituents of the skin: this is why over a long time ultraviolet radiation produces so much damage. This will be discussed in Chapter 4 ('Skin and ageing').

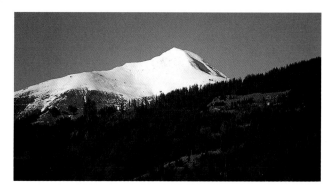

Sunlight reflected from snow – a damaging combination for our skin, since it contains a substantial proportion of ultraviolet radiation.

Prevention of water loss from the body

Throughout our lives our bodies naturally lose water by constant gentle evaporation through our skins (transepidermal water loss, TEWL), although we are unaware of the process. Preventing excessive water loss is exceptionally important in itself – both to the skin itself and to the body as a whole. In the normal epidermis the water content gets less the closer we get to the surface. Water makes up to 70–75% of the weight of the basal layer, but only 10–15% of the stratum corneum.

The stratum corneum is a particularly important barrier to the control of moisture loss.

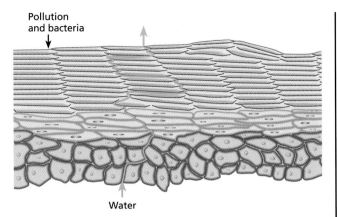

Pollution and bacteria

Water

The tightly packed cells of the stratum corneum (top) provide a barrier against harmful material from the outside world, as well as protection against water loss.

It is also a highly effective barrier against the outside environment, being tough but flexible *provided* it is well hydrated. If its water content falls below 10% it becomes dry, less flexible and increasingly prone to damage, breakdown and infection.

The epidermis as a whole is about 35 micrometres thick when dry, but can swell to 48 micrometres on full hydration. This depends more on the humidity and temperature of the surrounding air than on how much we have drunk!

SKIN MYTH

Drinking six or eight glasses of water a day will keep skin moisture levels high, and is an essential factor in renewing cells and hydrating the skin to prevent wrinkles from forming. It also helps to detoxify and remove waste.

Fact: Drinking more will not cause water to enter the skin selectively, unless the person is seriously dehydrated. Normal skin is well hydrated naturally. The excess water goes into all the tissues of the body, and ultimately to the bladder!

Detoxification of the body is carried out by organs such as the liver, which do not need vast amounts of water to function.

Preventing infection

The natural layer of oil-in-water emulsion on the skin is the first barrier against invasion by micro-organisms such as bacteria, fungi and yeasts. The stratum corneum provides the next level of defence.

White blood cells in the skin can capture and destroy bacteria invading the epidermis. As a result pus may form.

The epidermis also contains special defence cells (**Langerhans cells**) which are spread out amongst the keratinocytes. These cells mop up invading foreign substances that have found their way into the body, and take them off to special white cells (**lymphocytes**) in the lymph glands. Here they are neutralised.

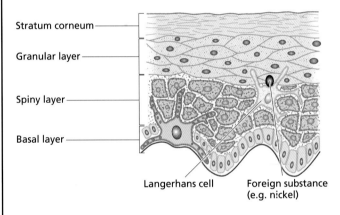

Stratum corneum

Granular layer

Spiny layer

Basal layer

Langerhans cell

Foreign substance (e.g. nickel)

A Langerhans cell in the skin.

An important element of defence concerns chemicals. If a chemical such as nickel is constantly absorbed through the skin, say from a button on one's jeans, it is first taken up by the Langerhans cells; later, however, special lymphocytes called **T-cells** make antibodies to that chemical. This can in time lead to an allergic skin reaction at the site of the button as the T-cells rush to meet the invading chemical. Allergies are discussed further in Chapter 9 ('The safety of cosmetic products').

Functions of the dermis

These include:

- giving mechanical protection to the body from bumps and knocks; the collagen has an important role in this function

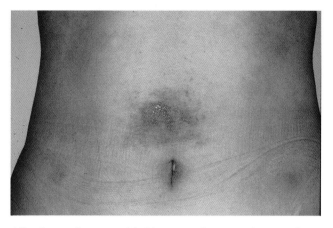

Allergic reaction to a nickel button – the Langerhans and T cells are responsible for this.

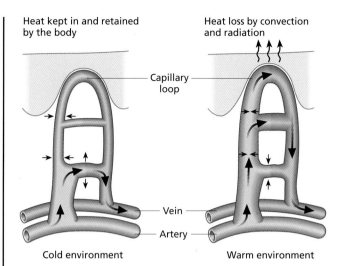

Heat kept in and retained by the body

Heat loss by convection and radiation

Capillary loop

Vein

Artery

Cold environment   Warm environment

Body temperature regulation by blood flow control: (left) blood vessels in the dermis get narrower when cold, so limiting the amount of heat brought by the blood to the skin surface and lost; (right) the vessels widen when warm, so that heat is brought to the surface and escapes.

- providing oxygen and nutrients, via blood in the tiny vessels that run in the ground substance, to the living part of the epidermis
- removing waste products of metabolism from the epidermis, which are also carried away in the blood
- providing shape and form to the body, by holding all its structures together
- contributing to skin colour, particularly in people with little melanin in the epidermis.

Organs in the dermis have special functions of their own:

- regulation of body temperature through control of blood flow and sweating
- skin sensations of touch, pain, heat and cold.

Sweating

One of the important functions of skin is in helping to control body temperature.

All primates (a group that includes apes and humans) have glands in the skin from which they produce sweat (see page 34) and control body temperature by evaporation (horses have them too). This sweat, which we don't notice, is called **insensible perspiration**. Evaporation needs heat energy, so evaporating sweat removes heat from the body and keeps down the body temperature (a process called **thermoregulation**). Sweat production is a response sometimes to external temperature changes, sometimes to internal stimuli – such as a highly seasoned curry! – and occasionally to

stress, as a reaction to increased production of adrenalin.

Control of body temperature through sweat production is essential for life. Unfortunately this mechanism encourages effects which are now considered unacceptable, such as excessive wetness and unpleasant markings on clothing, and body odour (malodour).

Most of the sweat produced by the body comes from the eccrine glands. Up to two litres can be lost in an hour! While its primary function is temperature control, eccrine sweat also provides a useful method of removing acids and some waste products (toxins) from the body.

Men sweat more than women do; on the other hand, women have a higher perspiration pH (pH 7) compared with men (pH 5.61).

Different skin types and their characteristics

As skin grows older, we start to see differences in its appearance – and not only differences in our own skins but differences between people of the same age. The changes are determined fundamentally by our inherited skin type, its response to its environment and sometimes our overall health.

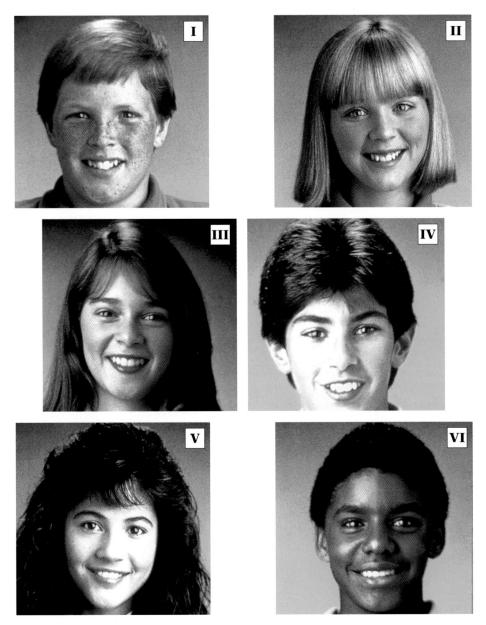

Classification of skin types

Human skin types

Skin type	Unexposed skin colour	Sun response
I	white	always burns, never tans
II	white	always burns, tans minimally
III	white	burns minimally, sometimes tans
IV	light brown	burns minimally, always tans well
V	brown	rarely burns, tans darkly (Asian skins)
VI	dark brown	never burns, tans darkly (African skins)

One way in which scientists define skin type is according to how it responds to exposure to the sun.

The system of classifying skin according to its type, shown in the table above, was developed on a two-factor basis: hair colour and the ability to tan. Classification under this system also indicates the people who are especially prone to develop skin cancer. The six-point scale is based on the answers people give when questioned about how they react to sun exposure.

Individuals who are types I and II have skin more likely to burn and have difficulty developing a tan. It is also these people who are at highest risk for the development of skin cancer. During the last two centuries or so, many people of this type have moved to sunny climates like those of Australia and South Africa and are now at a much higher risk of developing skin cancer than if they had stayed in Europe.

Skin type descriptions

Another way of classifying skin types becomes evident when people are asked to describe how *they* view their skins. For practical rather than necessarily scientific proposes, they will often describe their skin type as either normal, dry, greasy or mixed.

In the next part of this chapter we discuss each of these descriptions in turn.

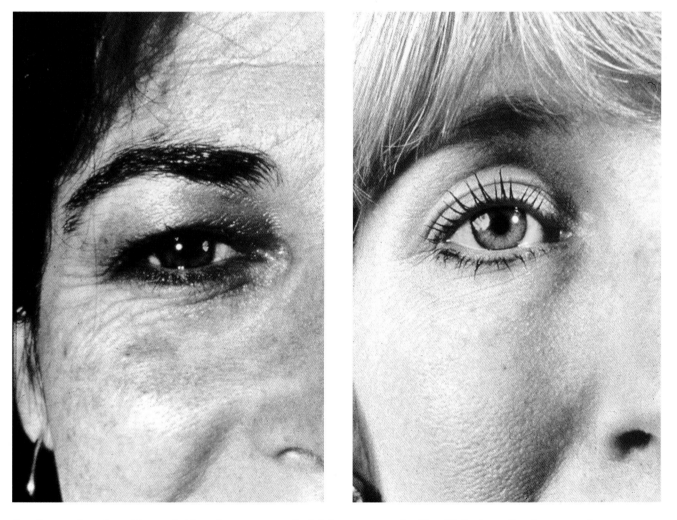

Sun damage in twins with type I skins: the woman on the left has spent much of her life in Australia, the one on the right in the UK.

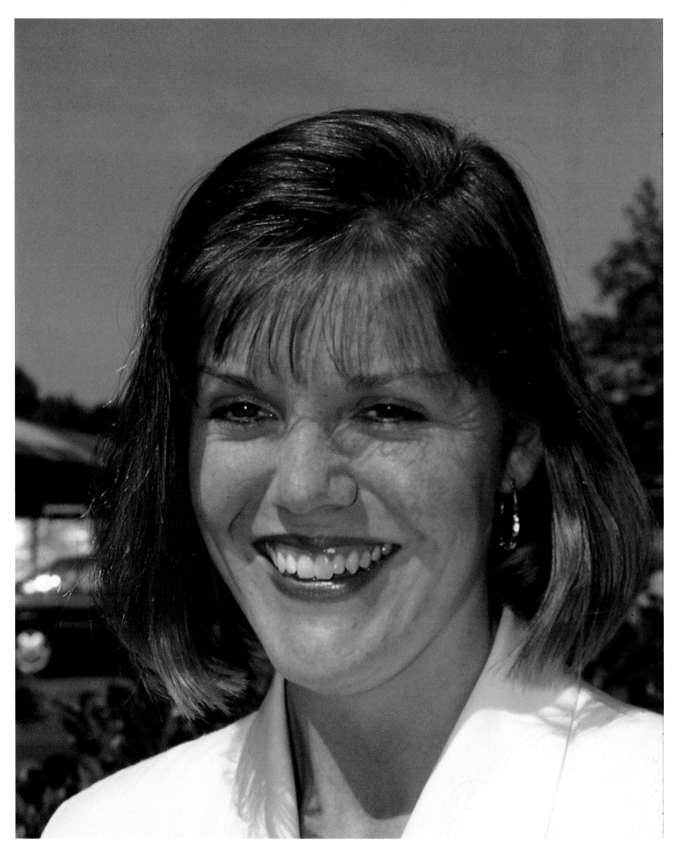

Normal skin that sometimes burns but eventually tans. Auburn hair and blue eyes are typical of north-western Europe and parts of the populations of countries such as North America, Australasia and South Africa. This type of skin is susceptible to the long-term effects of the sun.

Normal skin

The characteristics of so-called 'normal' skin can be summarised as follows:

- a clear appearance
- an even colour
- feels neither tight nor greasy
- soft and supple to the touch
- a high degree of elasticity.

Normal skin may be said to have nothing obviously wrong with it, and no sensations of discomfort. It results from a balance of the normal skin functions (including new skin cells being formed and old ones being lost, together with well-controlled water loss, sebum secretion and sweating). This creates a balanced state of suppleness, elasticity, colour and hue which is often characteristic of pre-adolescents.

Normal skin can quite quickly become 'abnormal', however. Failure to look after it, or abuse by sun, wind or cold, may lead to dry and damaged skin and ultimately the risk of premature development of lines and wrinkles.

Dry skin

Dry skin:

- feels tight and irritable
- often looks flaky
- often develops fine lines around the eyes
- tightens after washing with soaps or detergents or prolonged exposure to low humidity.

Dry skin is characterised most of all by this sensation of tightness, with the skin feeling rough and scaly and visible lines developing. At its worst it may look cracked. The problem lies in poor epidermal function and damage to the water/lipid barrier film, shown by an increase in the rate of transepidermal water loss (TEWL).

Patches of dry skin may arise from apparently normal skin, or sometimes even greasy skin, that has been temporarily dried out, whether by sunburn, or by exposure to extremes of climate (cold, heat, wind or dryness) or to chemicals such as detergents and solvents or to air conditioning. In young people the main problem of dry skin is a reduced production of sebum.

Dryness is a significant problem associated with mature skin as hydration ability progressively decreases and the skin's mechanical properties deteriorate, with loss of suppleness and flexibility.

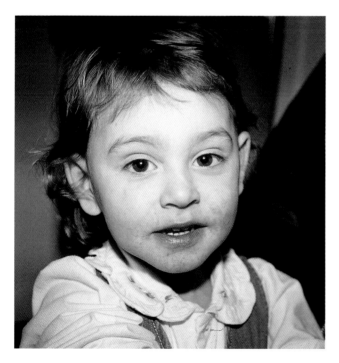

Dry skin can be troublesome (left) in children and equally (right) in old age – this skin is nearly 80 years old.

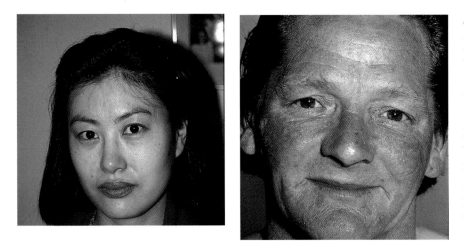

Greasy skin often develops at puberty but can persist into adulthood. The sebaceous glands are more prominent on the forehead, nasal areas and upper chest than on the lower half of the body.

Greasy (oily) skin

Greasy skin (sometimes called **seborrhoeic skin**) generally appears at puberty although in a few people it starts much earlier, from the age of six upwards. It is rare after the age of 35. It involves only the upper part of the body, where greater numbers of sebaceous glands are found.

This type of skin is particularly common in adolescents and young adults. At this age there is in both sexes a dramatic increase in sebum production under the influence of the male sex hormones. The extra sebum gives the skin a shiny appearance, especially on the nose and forehead. The epidermis tends to thicken, due to increased keratin production, and the pores dilate. As a result the skin feels rough and irregular.

Mixed skin

Mixed skin (often called **combination skin**) is characterised on the face by thickened, shiny skin associated with patches of dry skin.

Sensitive skin

In addition to these recognised types of skin, many people believe that they have 'sensitive skin'.

Doctors and scientists are not completely agreed about what 'sensitive skin' is, but it may generally be considered as skin which is easily irritated. It is more commonly associated with people with type I skin, and probably has a genetic element.

Some people with this condition cannot tolerate contact with any cosmetic products, however well-formulated they may be.

Sensitive skin can be associated with a medical condition called **atopy**, where people have an inherited predisposition to eczema, hay fever and asthma. Atopy is discussed further in Chapter 3, 'Some common skin problems'.

In several surveys, up to 70% of women said they thought they had 'sensitive skin'.

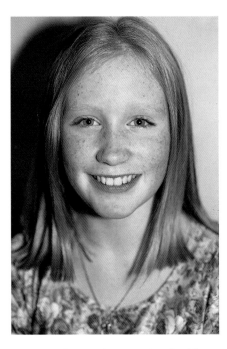

Sensitive skin is often associated with type I skin.

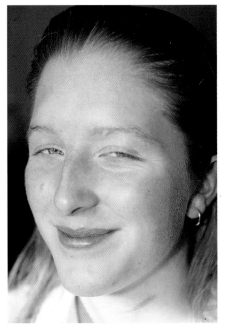

The transient reaction to shampoo of a highly 'sensitive' skin.

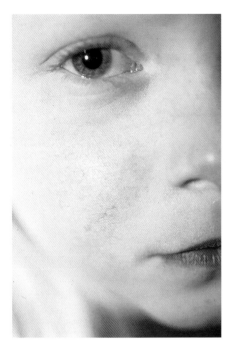

Atopic skin. About 15–20% of the population have the genetic ability to develop eczema, asthma and hay fever. The figure has risen considerably in the last few decades.

Truly sensitive or atopic skin may:

- feel very tight after washing
- have a naturally high TEWL rate
- react to many external stimuli by becoming red and blotchy
- be prone to developing dry flaky patches.

Variation with site on the body

Whatever the type of skin, its state and function will differ from one part of the body to another even in the same individual, and will change from time to time. For example, the face, forearms and hands are most exposed to the elements and may suffer from drying and cracking. The bottom is scarcely ever exposed and the skin there is almost always in near-perfect condition. To really see the differences in skin condition in one person, these are the two areas to examine!

Another characteristic that shows considerable variation is the density of the sebaceous glands. There are many more sebaceous glands per unit area of skin in the upper part of the body (forehead >300 per cm^2; chest 60 per cm^2; upper back 80 per cm^2).

Another example of a variable characteristic is the permeability of the skin: the skin of the palms of the hands is less permeable than that of the forearm, which in turn is less permeable than that of the scalp.

The rate at which the stratum corneum loses corneocytes as squames also depends on the body site. Squames are lost more rapidly from the forearm and back, for example, than from the upper arm and abdomen.

Factors affecting skin function

Environments that dehydrate the skin can considerably affect the skin condition, and hence its functions. Examples include centrally heated and air-conditioned homes and offices.

Out of doors, sun and wind together may produce very severe drying effects, especially if they are experienced over a long period of time.

Water and harsh household detergents and cleaning fluids are the most damaging factors of all, particularly to the hands. People who work as cleaners or apprentice hairdressers expose the skin of their hands to water and chemicals all day long, almost every day. This can result in chronically dry and chapped hands, which may result in a form of **irritant dermatitis** if left untreated. In turn they may become prone to develop allergies to products with which they come into contact, producing an **allergic dermatitis**. These conditions are discussed in more detail in Chapter 10, 'The safety of cosmetic products'.

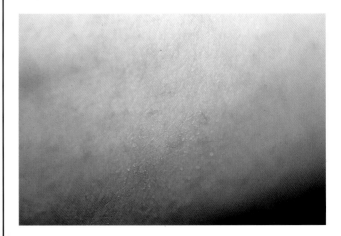

Reaction of dry skin to washing.

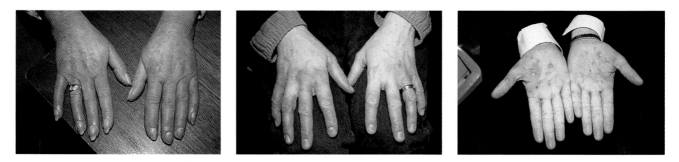

Irritant dermatitis (left); hand eczema I (middle and right). Three examples of the effect of the environment on skin function. In all three the chronic irritation leading ultimately to hand eczema here was due to the effects of water and harsh detergents.

Climate

Climate can make a considerable difference to the state of all our skins. Where we live in the world, and whether we are adapted to the local climate there, may also be critical.

The humidity of the air is important to the way we feel and how our skin condition fares. Humidity is largely determined by temperature: this is because the air can hold more water vapour at higher temperatures. In winter the air cannot hold as much water, and on a very cold day there is virtually no moisture in the air at all. This is why we can often see people's breath in frosty weather: as the warm, moist air from the lungs cools down, the water vapour in it turns into tiny liquid drops that form clouds.

In hot weather, most of us find dry air more comfortable and pleasant than very humid air. The tropics are hot and humid, while Scandinavia can be warm and dry. Many people find hot, humid weather trying and difficult to tolerate: this is the kind of weather in which, in certain countries, seems to accentuate a tendency for riots to break out! The skin, however, prefers humidity to dryness.

Skin condition in winter

The condition of skin can change from day to day, and even from hour to hour. It may be affected by general health, by changes in hormones during the menstrual cycle and by the immediate environment. Skin that felt normal in the morning may feel greasy and uncomfortable after a day spent travelling in crowded trains and working in an office with rather inefficient ventilation.

Skin needs to maintain water balance with the environment for ideal function. As we have seen, the epidermis, particularly the stratum corneum, acts as a partial water barrier, helping to regulate the amount of water in the skin. This barrier *itself* needs adequate water (more than 10%) to function properly.

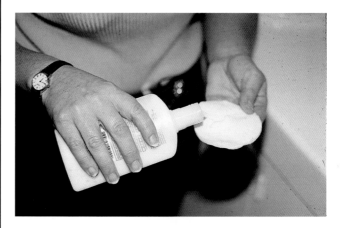

Cleaning the skin after a day's work reveals how much sebum and dirt was trapped in it. Much of this has to do with the amount of moisture in the environment and the level of pollution.

This water is used to ensure that the other vital part of the barrier, the lipid structures between the cells of the stratum corneum, is maintained in a fluid state. Damage to the stratum corneum – for example, by washing with harsh soaps, which removes both external and internal lipids – can disrupt this barrier and set up a 'vicious circle' of drying:

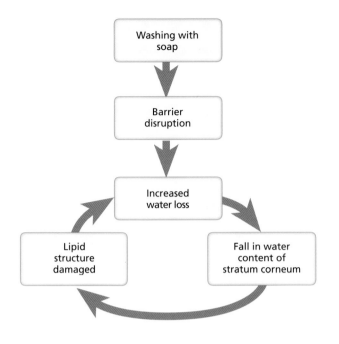

In fact, skin has to fight a daily battle against the drying effects of the environment.

But this drying effect is worse in the winter months. Although air in the winter months often feels damper, on average it has less *relative* humidity than in the summer – that is, humidity compared to that of the skin.

In winter the difference between the concentration of water in the air and that in the skin exerts a considerable drawing force on water in the skin. If the skin becomes drier, the lipid structure of the barrier tends to break up. As a result, water cannot be retained so easily. The cycle of water loss is set up again.

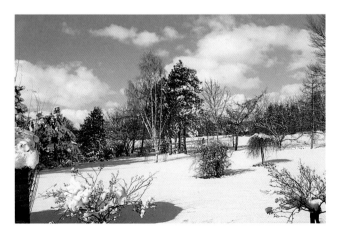

In the winter months, air has less relative humidity and the skin tends to dry more rapidly.

Another factor is that the stratum corneum simply doesn't like the cold. Cold makes keratin stiffer and less flexible – you will probably be familiar with the 'tight' feeling that skin has in the winter.

As a result of all these factors, skin tends to be drier and in worse condition in the winter months than at other times of the year. In extreme cases, this constant drying effect can lead to cracking, flaking and redness. In the winter, skin tends to lose the battle against the environment. That's when it needs to be looked after most.

In the winter, a moisturiser can be regarded as essential to maintain healthy skin – even so-called 'normal' skin. As we will see later, a moisturiser performs several important functions. It enables lost water to be replaced, and then helps to keep it in the skin by the **humectants** (water-binding agents) that it contains (see page 103). One such is glycerol. Scientists have shown that humectants play a vital role in the skin by helping to maintain the lipids of the epidermis in good condition, vital to its water-retaining properties.

A good moisturiser will deliver water to the skin effectively and keep it in the skin for as long as possible.

INGREDIENTS:
Aqua, PPG-15 stearyl ether, Glycerin, Stearyl alcohol, Salicylic acid, Cetyl betaine, Distearyldimonium chloride, Oxidised polyethylene, Sodium lauryl sulfate, Alcohol denat, Behenyl alcohol, BHT, Cetyl alcohol, Disodium EDTA, Menthol, Parfum, PPG 30, Sodium sulfate, Steareth 2, Steareth 21.

Glycerol (often called 'glycerin'), one of the best known humectants, is an ingredient of nearly all moisturisers.

Coming in from the cold
Coming into a warm room from the cold outdoors will often restore a rosy glow to the skin and soften it to some degree. This is due to the blood vessels in the skin opening up in the warmth.

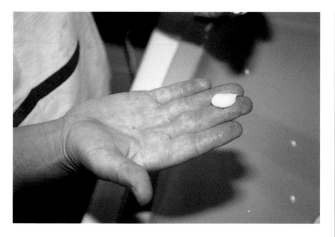

The use of moisturisers on both hands and face is especially important in winter.

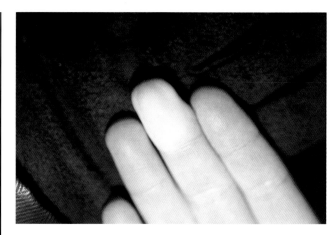

Raynaud's phenomenon: bleaching of the skin caused by sudden shut-down of blood vessels – prevent it by wearing gloves in cold weather.

This will *not* help to restore moisture, however. It may even encourage more water loss, since the air in centrally heated houses is often drier than that outside!

Sebum production in winter

Sebum (the lipid mixture produced by the skin's sebaceous glands, see page 34) is produced at a fairly constant rate in each individual, though rates vary from one person to another and tend to be higher overall in the teenage years. It does not change in response to time of day or season, though sebum will obviously build up on the skin throughout the day. (This is why skin feels sticky at the end of the day.)

Since sebum production is neither significantly lower or higher in the winter, there is no need to use a moisturiser with extra (or less) 'grease' in the winter to compensate for a lack (or excess) of sebum.

Skin appearance in winter

As we have seen (page 10), the skin's response to cold is to close down the small blood vessels in the dermis. This diverts blood from the surface of the body to the inside, and helps to check heat loss.

The result can be that in cold weather skin loses the glow it normally gains from blood flow close to the surface, and it can tend to look dull and lifeless. Massaging with a moisturiser will help to stimulate circulation near the surface and give the skin more colour, as well as improving the water content. You can do this as often as you need to – you can't over-moisturise!

Some people have a particular sensitivity to even slight drops in the air temperature, resulting in the ends of their fingers going white. This is called **Raynaud's phenomenon**: although it can be painful it is otherwise harmless.

The essentials of winter skin care

- Use a good moisturising product during the day – it doesn't need to be a heavy cream, but it does need to hydrate well. Use it liberally and often.
- At night, use a good night cream. Night creams are specially formulated with a higher lipid content than would normally be comfortable in the day, to help restore softness to the skin.
- Do not wash with harsh soaps. Soaps dry the skin and exaggerate the effects of the cold. Use a good-quality mild cleanser formulated for 'sensitive' skin.
- Stay warm! Keep well wrapped up, to help maintain a soft skin by preventing excessive TEWL.

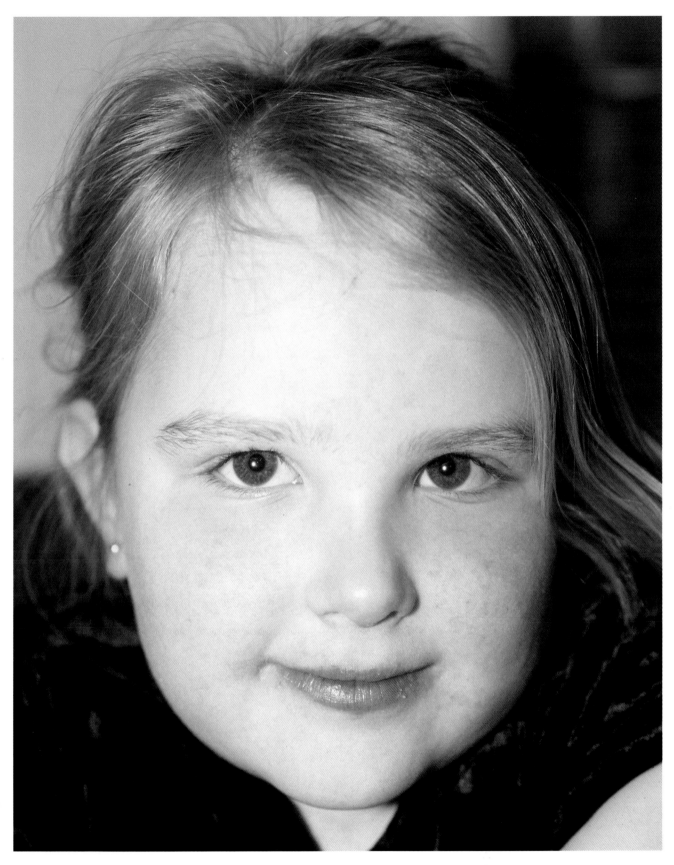

Dry, atopic skin like this is especially vulnerable to winter weather. Protection by generous and frequent application of moisturiser is vital.

Eczema on the eyelids...

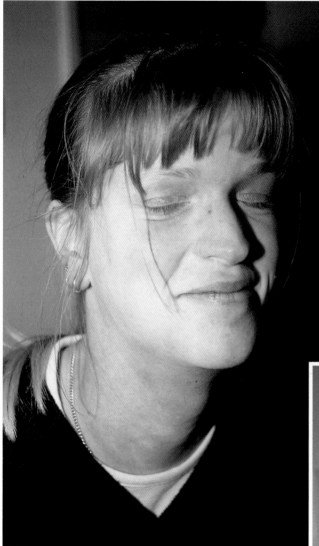

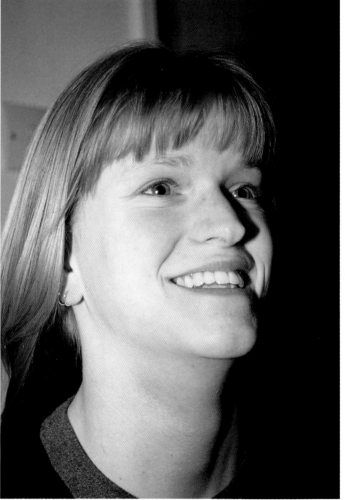

...can be treated with regular moisturising.

3

Some common skin problems

We all recognise that not everybody has beautifully clear skin. Some have dry and blotchy skin. Others have blemishes, too much pigment, or too little. In this chapter we describe some common skin problems that you may encounter.

Atopy

About 20% of the population have the inherited condition called **atopy**, which can lead to various degrees of dry skin or even eczema. People with this problem need to take extra care of their skin.

Atopic skin tends to have a higher than average TEWL and loses water readily. It can be very sensitive to irritants.

No one knows the precise cause of atopy, except that it has a genetic component: 70% of patients with atopic dermatitis have at least one relative who suffers from either eczema, asthma or hay fever.

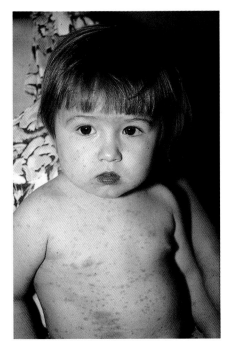
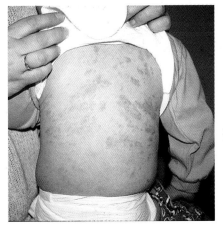
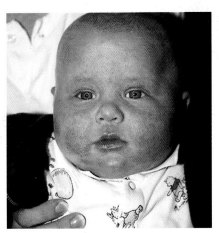

Atopy: 20% of the population have this condition, which is associated with a tendency to dry skin, eczema, hay fever and asthma.

Atopic eczema

Atopic eczema is becoming steadily more common. Among those born before 1960 the reported frequency is only about 2%, but it rises to between 9 and 20% in those born after 1970. The reason for the increase is still a mystery: it may be a real effect due to living in a more protected environment, or simply the result of better recognition of the condition, or perhaps both. Eczema is common among small children. It is often suggested that the cause may be diet intolerance, but this is probably rarely so.

Treatment

A family doctor can advise on managing eczema, but long-term commitment to skin care will be needed. Eczematous skin requires *constant* moisturising, and harsh soaps should be avoided. Careful use of steroid creams on the body may be helpful, but these products should only be used under medical supervision.

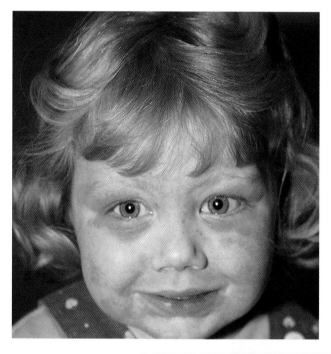

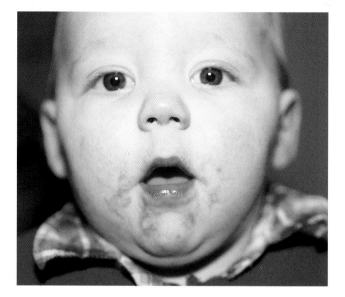

Eczema is made worse by scratching, and the facial eczema that is common among babies and toddlers is also worsened by dribbling.

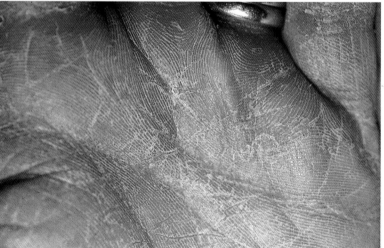

Hand eczema is very common, and is often associated with occupational diseases. In certain countries people with atopy are not permitted to take up hairdressing.

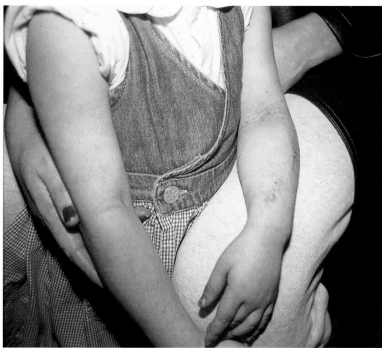

In childhood eczema the dry and cracked skin often appears in the creases of the elbows, knees and bottom – the so-called flexural eczema.

In adults, eczema tends to form patches.

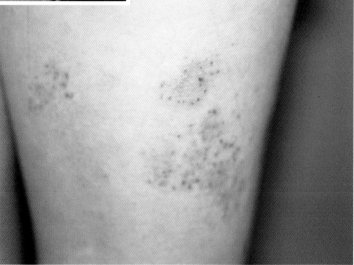

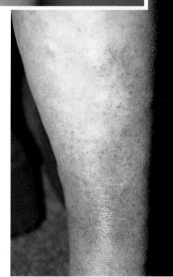

In elderly people eczema can be associated with poor circulation in the legs: this is known as varicose eczema.

Acne

Acne can affect all age groups, from a few months after birth to old age. During puberty, virtually all boys and 90% of girls will have some spots and pimples, which are usually mild forms of acne; nearly 85% of people aged between 12 and 25 will have had some acne.

The psychological effects of acne can be severe in some people, who may feel disfigured and unattractive because of the eruptions on their skin.

Many factors are concerned in the development of acne, including a hereditary predisposition and the presence of male hormones (in both boys and girls), which leads to increased sebum production and the presence on the skin of otherwise harmless bacteria called *Proprionibacterium acnes*. These multiply deep in the hair follicle and produce inflamed pus-filled spots.

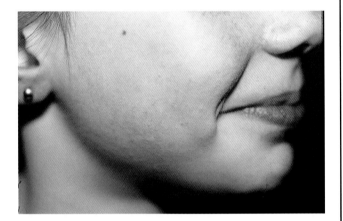

The early stages of acne: start using a specialised cleanser every day.

Treatment for acne

Prevention is better than cure!

The main aim of the treatment of acne is to *prevent* new spots appearing on the skin. Getting rid of existing spots is much more difficult: people having treatment are often disappointed because their spots don't disappear quickly. Acne sufferers need a great deal of patience!

A regular cleansing routine using specially formulated products (available from pharmacists and retail outlets) can help to remove surface sebum and the bacteria associated with acne. If these products are conscientiously used on a daily basis they can help to reduce the number of spots that will occur in the future.

People who already have mild to moderate acne should use products specifically formulated for this condition: these contain special ingredients for the prevention of spots, such as salicylic acid or benzoyl peroxide, which remove

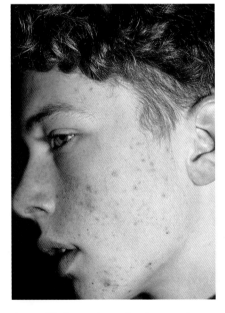

Acne affects most people at some stage around puberty, but it can be controlled.

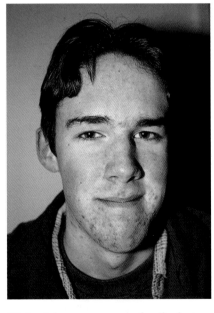

Moderately severe acne: a family doctor will be able to help.

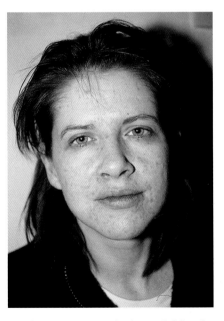

Rarely, acne can persist into adulthood: this sufferer is 35 years old.

SKIN MYTHS ABOUT ACNE

Chocolate and fatty foods cause acne.

Fact: This is just one of the many myths about diet and acne. It is true that acne is less common in some countries where diets are markedly different from ours, but this difference may be due to genetic factors. There is little scientific evidence to indicate that diet plays a significant role in the development of acne.

Sunlight exposure improves acne.

Fact: There is no conclusive evidence to show ultraviolet radiation improves acne. A tan may mask erythema (reddening of the skin) and provide some cosmetic improvement.

Poor hygiene causes acne.

Fact: If acne were caused by a lack of soap and water, it would probably occur between the toes. In fact, too much scrubbing and friction aggravate acne.

Acne is a disease that mainly affects teenagers.

Fact: Many adults have acne or acne variants: the condition can even occur for the first time in elderly people.

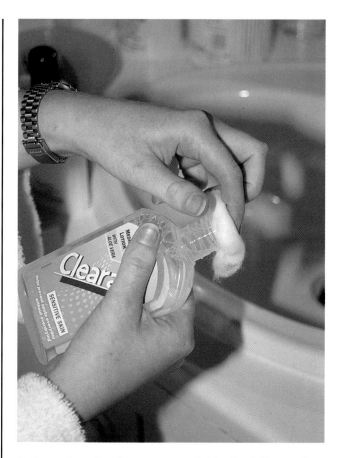

Spots can be reduced or even prevented by the daily use of a specialist product.

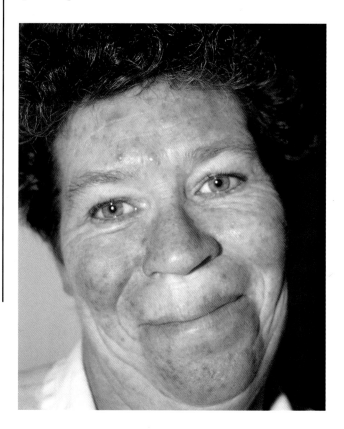

keratin and kill the bacteria. These will provide a treatment that can help to reduce the number of existing spots on the skin.

In cases of persistent or severe acne a doctor should always be consulted: effective treatments are available, but only with medical supervision.

Rosacea was formerly known as 'acne rosacea', but is not ▶ related to the teenage condition. It can be controlled by medication from a dermatologist or experienced family doctor. It is not caused by excessive alcohol, although this can make it look worse as the blood vessels dilate.

Other common skin problems

The following series of photos and descriptions shows some others of the more common skin disorders, which may be medical or cosmetic, together with an indication of what remedies (if any) may be helpful. We all see these conditions in our own skin, or that of others, from time to time.

▶ *A cold sore* is an eruption on the margin of the lips. It is caused by the virus herpes simplex, which lives in the body and escapes the immune system. Cold sores develop when the skin is damaged during a cold or after sunbathing. They can be suppressed by anti-viral creams available from pharmacists, but usually they die out even if untreated.

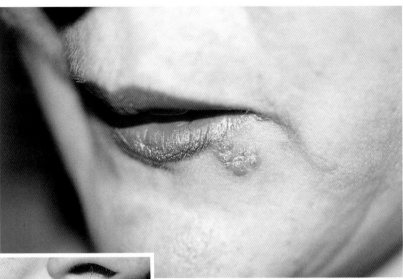

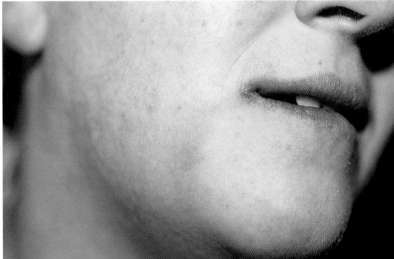

◀ *Angular cheilosis* takes the form of small splits at the side of the mouth, made worse by licking. The cause is unknown, although the condition is often (wrongly) attributed to vitamin deficiency. It is eased by using lip salve frequently.

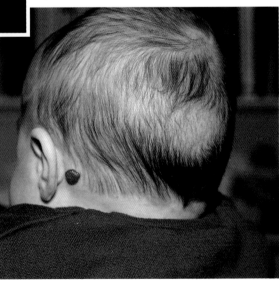

▶ This scarlet bleb is a **haemangioma**, a harmless collection of dilated blood vessels. It can be dealt with easily by a doctor.

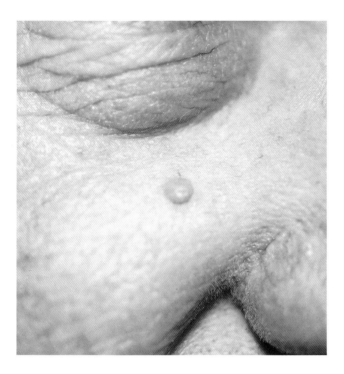

◄ ***Warts*** *are very common. They are caused by viruses that normally live happily on the skin surface but penetrate the stratum corneum when it is damaged. They are most often seen on the fingers and the feet (when they are usually called veruccas). They can be treated by creams available from pharmacies, or by freezing.*

▶ ***Seborrhoeic warts*** *are raised pigmented spots associated with ageing: they are not caused by viruses or by cancers, and are quite harmless. If they become unsightly they can be scraped off by a dermatologist.*

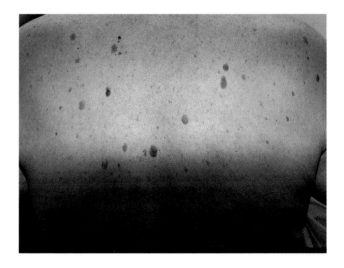

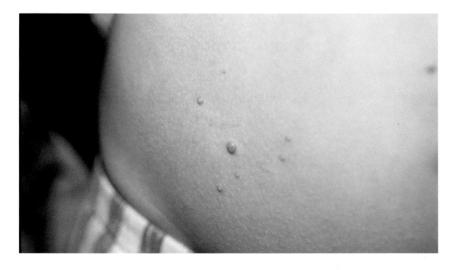

◄ ***Molluscum contagiosum*** *is common in children and is caused by a harmless virus. It is seen as rapidly spreading spots, rather like a chicken pox rash. No treatment is necessary as the spots disappear spontaneously.*

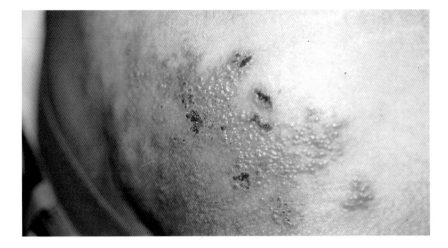

◄ **Shingles** is a very common condition that is caused by the chicken pox virus, which lives on in everyone who has had the disease. It erupts in this typical line on the trunk or the face. Contrary to the popular myth, it is not contagious.

► **Chicken pox**: these are the intensely irritating 'blisters' characteristic of this common childhood infection. It is probably not contagious for more than a day or two after the spots appear. There is no specific treatment other than to prevent scratching by applications of calamine lotion, to avoid damaging the dermis with consequent lifelong scarring.

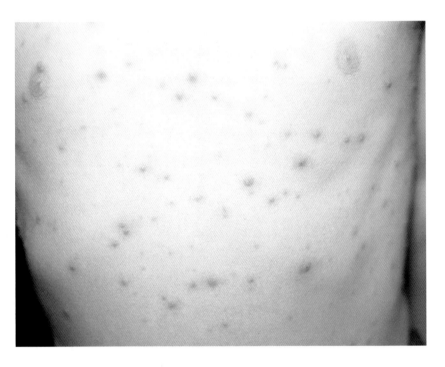

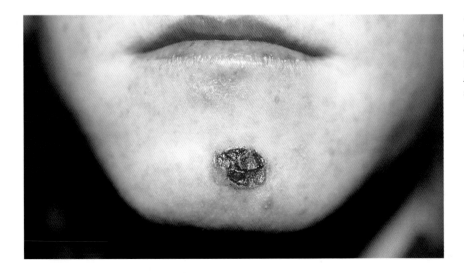

◄ **Impetigo**: a superficial skin infection, often seen around the mouth, nose and chin, especially in children. It is not necessarily due to poor hygiene. Antibiotics can be prescribed by a doctor and will cure it rapidly.

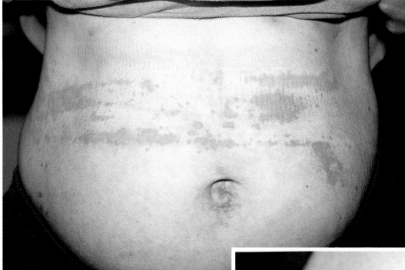

Urticaria, or 'nettle rash', is often associated with allergy since it looks like a reaction to stinging nettles. It forms acutely itchy swollen patches on the skin, which usually subside quickly although occasionally it becomes chronic. It can be caused by reaction to penicillin, certain foods, sunlight or even stress; it is sometimes caused by pressure from a tight garment, which is why it is often falsely attributed to washing powder residues in clothing.

It can be treated by anti-histamine tablets or, if very severe, by steroids prescribed by a doctor.

Psoriasis: a common skin condition which is due to over-production of cells in the epidermis with incomplete desquamation: this is what causes the heaped-up skin areas and scaly patches. It is essential to get a doctor's advice.

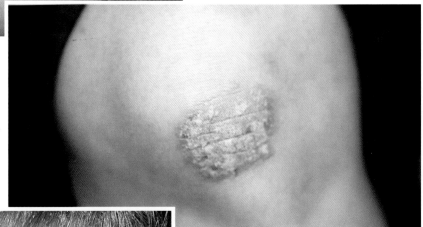

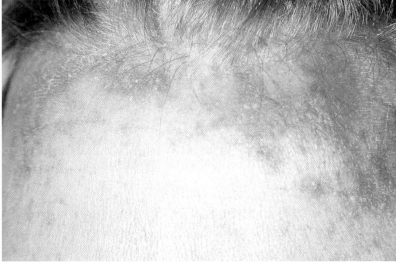

▲ The cause of the greasy scales and crusts of **seborrhoeic dermatitis** is unknown, but it is known to be a form of chronic eczema and psoriasis. It commonly occurs in the hair line, and affects beards and eyebrows too. It may lead to infections: medical advice is necessary.

▼ *Cradle cap* is an excessive desquamation resembling eczema. In infants it clears spontaneously, but in older children it may need treatment with special shampoo.

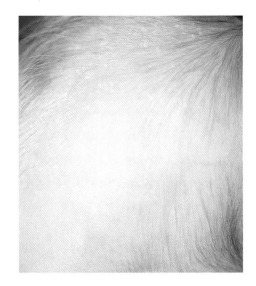

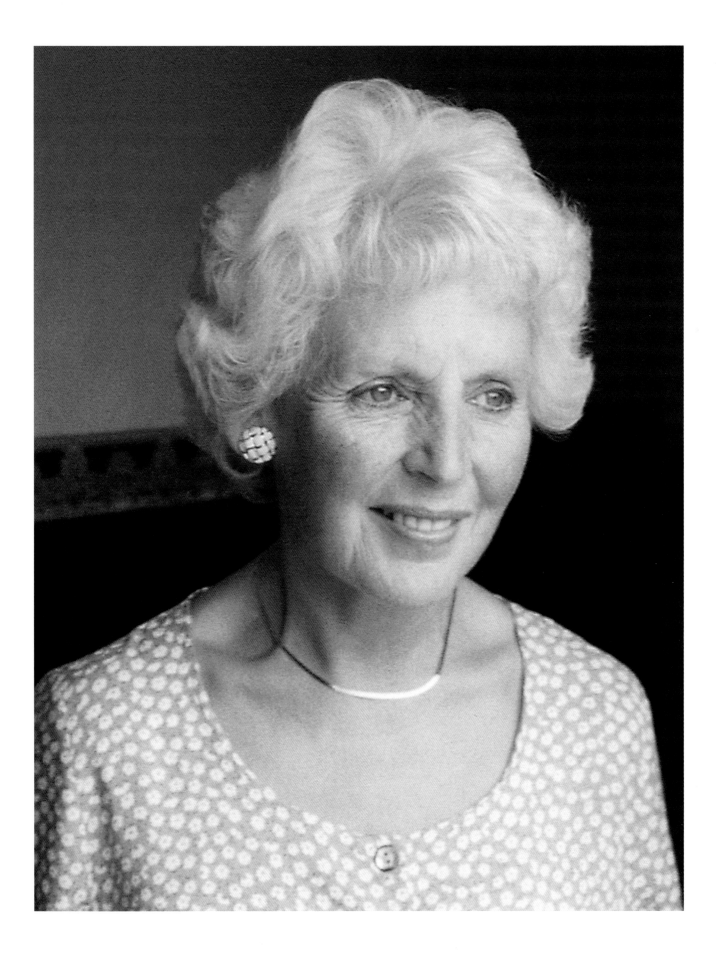

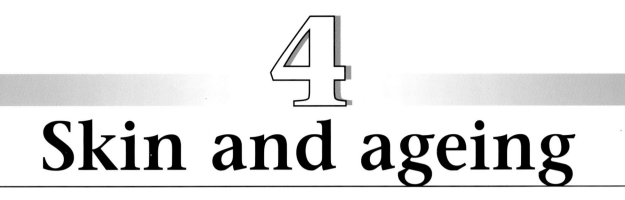

4
Skin and ageing

Nothing can alter the passage of time. But it is not just time that affects our skin. The age an individual *appears* to be depends on many factors. The genes are important, but even more crucial is the way the skin and body are treated throughout life. When we say some one is in the 'bloom of youth' it is usually because the skin exudes a certain kind of radiance and vitality. For most of us this tends to diminish naturally over time: from our skin's point of view at least, nothing is as good as pre-adolescence.

Scientists can explain this. What we call 'radiance' is a visual effect, mostly from the face, which implies a perfectly normal well-functioning skin. When the bloom fades it is because the skin begins to lose its ability to retain moisture. It becomes drier and more flaky, and shows the results of exposure to the environment, accumulated over many years. If we say someone has 'good skin', it often means that that person

was lucky in the lottery of gene inheritance, has been able to protect and look after the skin well, and that it has not changed as much since childhood as has that of others.

In former times only the 'idle rich' could concentrate on caring for their skins. Until this century most other people in the world worked on the land and were exposed to the elements. This is no longer true for most people in the developed countries.

How skin changes with age

Changes in skin appearance

We all know that as we get older, there can be dramatic changes in the way our skin looks.

The reasons why the skin of a child looks so healthy (at least, before the teenage spots come) are that the epidermis is highly translucent, it works very efficiently, and it easily retains water. More importantly, at this age there has been little or no obvious damage to the dermis

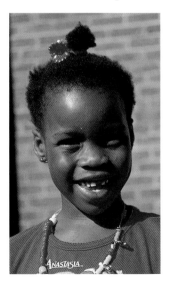
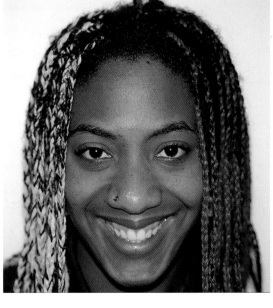
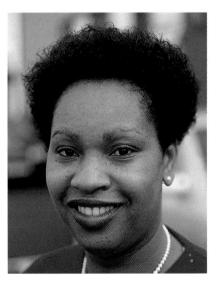

'Radiance' is the optical effect of light reflected from an undamaged dermis and well-organised epidermis. As we age our skin, if well looked after and protected from the sun, may be preserved better than that of our peers. Higher levels of pigment in the skin help to protect it but are not a total safeguard.

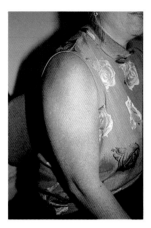
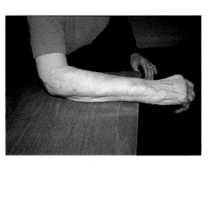
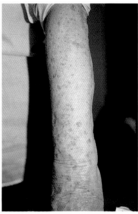

The appearance of the skin can change dramatically with age.

from the effects of the sun (although this is the time when most of the damage is being done and its effects will start to become visible within a few years).

As we grow out of childhood our skin naturally changes. During the teenage years hormonal changes account for an increase in sebum secretion and the development of spots and acne. Later in life, this extreme hormone production declines.

As we age, the rate of loss of the old skin cells from the stratum corneum slows down.

As well as this, the epidermis gradually gets less translucent and does not retain water so well. All the skin functions take place more slowly in mature skin. In addition, as most of us have been exposed to the sun to a greater or lesser degree over many decades, the 'damage' to the dermis can now be seen even through the dry epidermis.

This is why older skin looks dry, less radiant and less plumped out. This affects all races, but those who deliberately avoid the sun will tend to preserve their skins for longer.

The rate at which our skin changes is dependent to some extent on what we inherited in the first place, how we treated it and how we looked after it. The effect of ageing on skin is one of the features of skin that trouble us most. Our anxiety about its aspects has led to a whole industry setting out to prevent and correct the damage we do to ourselves over many years.

Intrinsic and extrinsic ageing

Some of the skin changes that accompany ageing are natural and inevitable, and together make up the process called **intrinsic ageing** or sometimes **chronological ageing**.

More significant for most people are the changes arising from external causes – called **extrinsic ageing** – and in particular the damage caused by ultraviolet radiation from the sun and sun beds, known as **photoageing**.

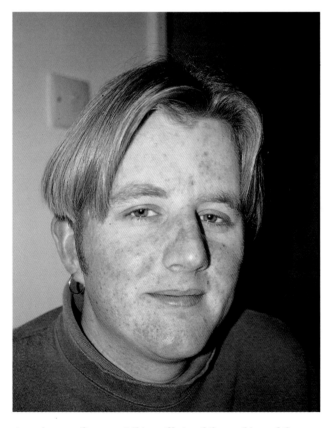

Acne is one of many striking effects of the peaking of the sex hormones at puberty.

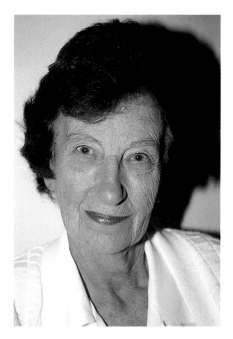

(left) Intrinsic ageing: this lady's skin is relatively clear but has lost much of its elastic properties. She has avoided the sun for most of her life.

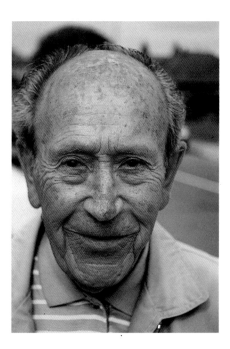

(right) A lifetime's exposure produces all the features of photoageing, including dull skin (due to a thickened epidermis) and a disorganised dermis. Service abroad in the armed forces is a major factor in the photodamage experienced by this age group.

These changes affect the dermis in particular and result from changes in the chemical structure of the collagen and elastin, and to the quality and quantity of proteins and natural acids in the skin.

Understanding the changes that occur in the cells and layers of the skin with intrinsic and extrinsic ageing will help us to understand why skin looks as it does, and how we can protect or alter this appearance. It also allows us to understand why it is so important to protect the skin of children and to educate them in skin care.

In **intrinsic ageing**, the skin becomes thinner and loses much of its elasticity, while the normal expression lines deepen. The boundary between the epidermis and the dermis is flattened, and the dermis starts to wither (atrophy). The number of blood vessels in the dermis begins to fall. At the same time the hair often loses its colour, and within the skin there are fewer hair follicles and fewer sweat glands. The collagen, elastin and ground substance also decrease in amount, but the proteins remain in a reasonably stable state.

In **extrinsic ageing** the epidermis thickens. The amounts of collagen and elastin increase, but the structures of these proteins become disorganised. Almost all of this is due to effects of radiation from the sun, known as **photodamage**.

■ *'Intrinsic ageing' happens inevitably.*

■ *'Extrinsic ageing' is due to outside factors that have affected the skin.*

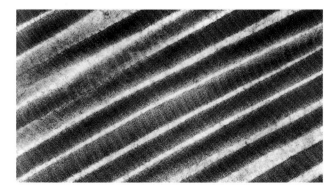

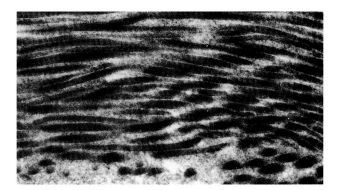

The collagen network from (left) undamaged and (right) sun-damaged skins.

Skin ageing in men and women

The processes of ageing differ in male and female skin.

In men, there is a gradual thinning of male skin with increasing age of approximately 1% per year. On the other hand the thickness of most women's skins remains surprisingly constant until the menopause, after which there is a significant and sometimes dramatic thinning with increasing age.

There is a relationship between skin thickness and collagen content in men of all ages. A similar relationship exists among women over 60 years of age, but it is less evident in younger women.

In adult skin, the features of ageing are closely related to the total collagen content, which in both sexes decreases with increasing age, but at different rates. In later life women may look older than men of the same age and similar experience of sun exposure, partly because their skin has a lower collagen content to start with. Another reason for the sex difference in skin collagen content may be the difference in male hormone production between men and women.

In women, oestrogen and androgen output from the ovaries and adrenal glands falls after menopause, resulting in decreased collagen synthesis and repair.

Ageing related to the failure of oestrogen production at the menopause accentuates intrinsic ageing, and together with photoageing may dramatically increase the apparent age of a menopausal woman.

Oestrogen deficiency particularly affects the fibroblasts of the dermis, and thinning of the skin is primarily related to a decrease in the production of collagen. This decrease is related

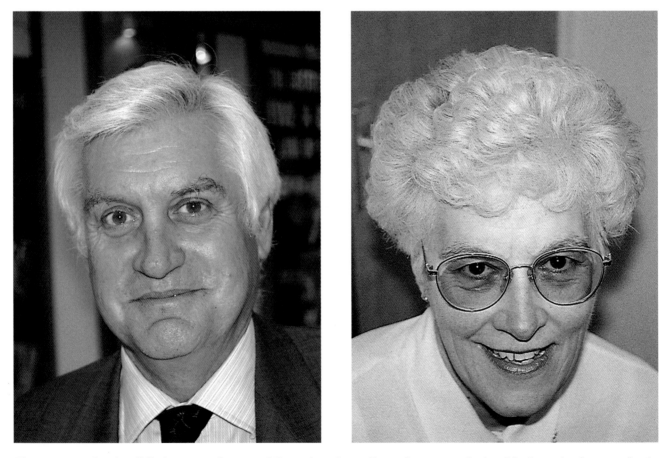

The processes of ageing differ in men and women. Women have less collagen than men to begin with. A man's sebaceous glands are active well into his 80s, whereas a woman's tend to stop functioning at the menopause, with the decline of oestrogen. Oestrogen deficiency and oestrogen replacement are major factors in women's skin health as well as in general health.

to a decline of bone mineral content with age, which can lead to the condition of osteoporosis. The fibroblasts are also responsible for the synthesis of the dermis ground substance, particularly glycoproteins and hyaluronic acid (which is able to bind water). The decrease in fibroblast activity with age accounts for the decreased dermal hydration.

Skin elasticity decreases with age, but the effect is more marked in women than in men.

In the epidermis, a lack of oestrogen slows down the activity of the basal keratinocytes, and consequently leads to epidermal atrophy. This atrophic fragile skin is less well protected by the normal surface film of lipids, because of the slow decline in sebum secretion experienced by everyone as they age. The stratum corneum barrier is less effective, and the skin may develop reactions to irritants, particularly if skin care has been inadequate or too aggressive.

Regular daily protection against the sun from an early age, combined with the regular use of well-formulated moisturisers, is of the greatest importance to 'preserving' the skin.

How skin changes with age: a summary

Age	Appearance	Physiology
<15	Nearly perfect skin. Smooth texture, pores small.	Excellent repair capabilities. Low sebaceous gland activity. Skin hydration good.
15–25	Acne key factor in surface texture. Fine lines start to appear, pore size increasing.	High sebaceous gland activity. Mild drop in dermal repair, immune system and collagen synthesis. Strong cohesion between skin layers and rapid cell turnover. Small drop in skin hydration, noticed particularly in winter.
25–45	More fine lines and appearance of first wrinkles (photodamage). Early signs of sagging near the eye. Some loss of elasticity. Adult acne.	Moderate decrease in dermal repair, resulting in less collagen and increasing accumulation of damaged corrective tissue. Noticeable and significant drop in skin hydration.
45–55	More wrinkles, rough texture. Sallow yellow colour begins to appear. Pores and age spots enlarge and define. Sagging near eye and cheek.	Significant decrease in dermal repair and immune system. Continued dermal degradation. Cohesion between skin layers continues to decline. Thinning of epidermis and stratum corneum. Skin tends now to be dry.
55+	Wrinkles and fine lines in abundance. Uneven colour, pigmentation. Sagging worsens. Dark circles under eye.	Compromised dermal repair, abundance of damaged connective tissue. Low production of collagen and sebum. Increased local over-production of melanin.

Apparent age

Although the skin is itself a protection against radiation, this protection brings with it consequences of its own, leading to an 'apparent age' that is greater than one's real age.

The appearance of an individual's face and hands are often used as a rapid measure of age. Comparing the appearance of the face and forearms with that of less exposed areas demonstrates the major differences between intrinsic and photoaged skin.

Skin creases and lines

The differences in skin surface markings between young and mature skin that has always been protected are only slight. In the older skin there will have been some natural loss of collagen and elastin, but no other significant damage.

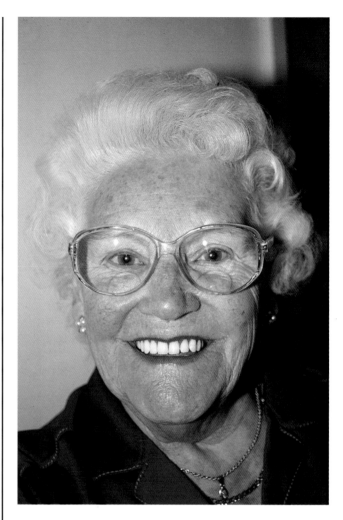

Photodamage to the skin of the face and the forearms increases one's apparent age.

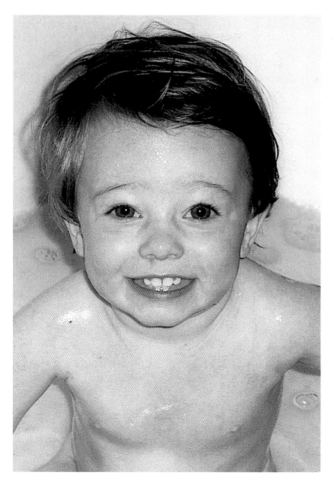

A young baby has the normal skin creases on the hands and face, but very few elsewhere on the body.

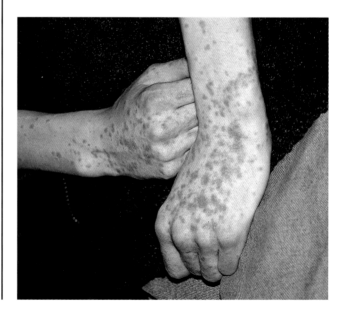

LINES AND WRINKLES

Fine lines are shallow grooves in the epidermis. They can be made to look less obvious by the use of cosmetic products that improve hydration and suppleness.

Wrinkles are of two types. The first is a **permanent** type that presents as a deep wrinkle on sun-exposed skin, such as the face and neck, and does not disappear on stretching.

The other type is a fine, shallow wrinkle that develops on sun-protected skin, such as the abdomen and bottom; this type of skin, becomes thin and wrinkles easily as the subcutaneous fat tissue decreases with age. These wrinkles disappear easily on stretching and so are **non-permanent**.

Cosmetic products cannot reverse wrinkle development. Wrinkles are effects of changes in the dermis, and cosmetics hardly reach the dermis at all.

There is no justification for the claims that certain cosmetic products containing collagen can put it back into the dermis. Collagen acts as a moisturiser in such products, but they do not replace what the skin has lost. Certain drugs such as isotretinoin (only available on a doctor's prescription) may stimulate collagen production when taken over many months, thus reducing the effects of sun damage to some extent.

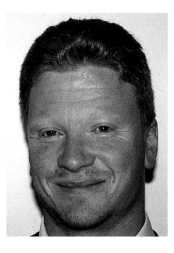

As we get older fine lines and wrinkles inexorably develop, mostly due to sun damage. This man has type I (Celtic) skin and must avoid the sun as much as possible.

As we grow older, fine lines and wrinkles begin to develop. The skin loses its firmness and elasticity. Expression lines form on the face, and patches of discoloration and areas of dilated blood vessels appear. On exposed areas of aged skin, the skin patterns are often markedly changed. Some very old people may find deep furrows develop in their skin. Others suffer from the so-called 'chicken neck'. The reasons for these changes are:

- blood circulation slows down
- metabolism slows down
- chemical changes take place in the tissues
- sebaceous glands diminish in size and number, particularly in women
- collagen production breaks down
- hormone production is altered or reduced.

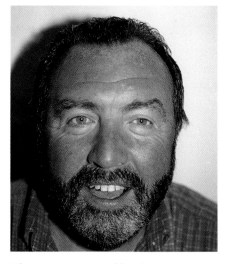

The permanent wrinkles due to sun damage do not disappear on stretching.

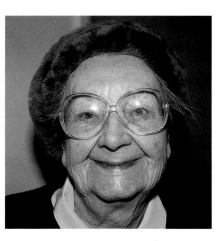

Wrinkles steadily increase in number and deepen with age – this lady is 92.

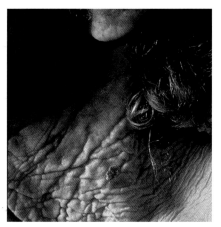

'Chicken neck'.

With increasing age, the skin's cell renewal process becomes less efficient. Tissue repair and cell regeneration slow down. The amount of natural moisture present in the skin is reduced. Because collagen production is less, the skin becomes thinner and loses its flexibility.

Changes in the protective function

The most obvious sign of intrinsic ageing is a decrease in the overall thickness of the epidermis as a whole, with a reduction in the number of cell layers. The number of cells in the stratum corneum does not diminish with age, however; this is important, because of the vital role of this layer as the skin barrier. On the other hand, the numbers of melanocytes and other cells do decrease with age. So do the numbers of the **Langerhans cells**, which are involved in the body's response to allergens (see page 40). This could be one reason why people tend to experience fewer allergic reactions as they get older.

The rete pegs become less prominent, and the junction of the dermis and epidermis becomes flattened (see page 10). This means that the epidermis is not so securely held down, and becomes more vulnerable to damage by friction.

Metabolism in the skin (as everywhere else) slows down. So too does the rate at which epidermal cells are produced, which may interfere with wound healing. The time necessary to repair the stratum corneum barrier increases considerably with age: the replacement of skin cells takes about twice as long for people over 75 as for those around 30.

Although the sebaceous glands themselves do not change much with increasing age, sebum production declines in many older people, especially after the age of 70, though in some the glands on the face actually enlarge in extreme old age.

With age, the number of active sweat glands falls and their output of sweat decreases too. As a result, perspiration is less in elderly skin. This explains why older people often find it hard to adapt to hot weather.

Most older people have a dry skin and therefore have a special need to avoid the over-use of harsh soaps and detergents, in order to prevent problems associated with dryness. Aged

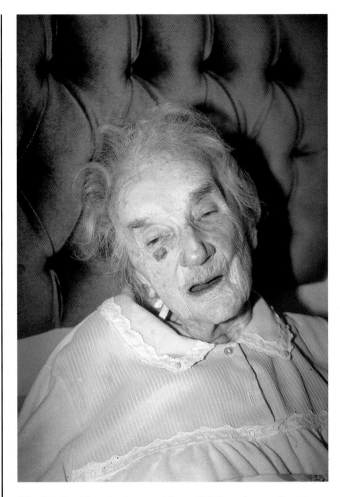

The fragile skin of extreme old age (103) no longer functions well. Subcutaneous fat and muscle have both deteriorated.

skin retains its fundamental ability to control water loss, but may partially lose this ability if the stratum corneum barrier becomes damaged by physical or chemical agents. Many substances will penetrate aged skin more easily than young skin.

The sun

The sun is the source of all life on Earth. Heat, light and warmth from the solar furnace sustain us all. There is a price to pay, however: the cumulative effects of invisible rays on our skin.

In parts of the world where the sun is very strong the local people usually avoid exposure, particularly when the sun is high in the sky. For example, people in tropical Africa do not stay out of doors for long if they can help it. Many of them feel uncomfortable in the sun's glare, complaining of feeling unbearably hot, possibly because of the vast heat production by the free radicals formed.

In some parts of Asia and Africa, a dark skin is considered unenviable, and a mark of lower social class. (This is because even dark skin can respond to sun exposure by tanning or by forming isolated areas of hyperpigmentation – that is, excessive pigment production – and so might be thought to denote an outdoor occupation: as in many societies, outdoor workers tend to have a lower status than office employees.) Many Asian women wear make-up to help the skin on the face and chest look paler, seeing this as a mark of higher social class. Some African women use powerful drugs and chemicals to lighten their skin for the same reason, occasionally with horrifying effects.

Health effects of sunlight

A whole travel industry was founded on people's desire to get away from more miserable climates to the sun, and to acquire a tan at almost any cost. Yet this very sunlight is potentially damaging to the skin in the short term and a significant health hazard in the long term – the actual benefits of sun exposure are few indeed.

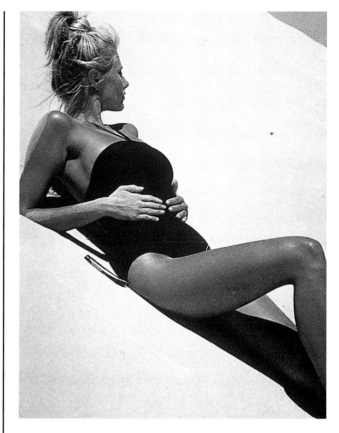

The sun is dangerous when transmitted from a blue sky in the middle of the day in summer or at high altitude. Remember – if you can see the blue, the blue can see you!

Noël Coward was right: it truly is only 'mad dogs and Englishmen who go out in the mid-day sun'.

Pigmentation changes are not uncommon in Asian people with chronically photodamaged skin. Such changes are especially clearly seen in the man on the left, who was a plantation worker in south-east Asia for many years.

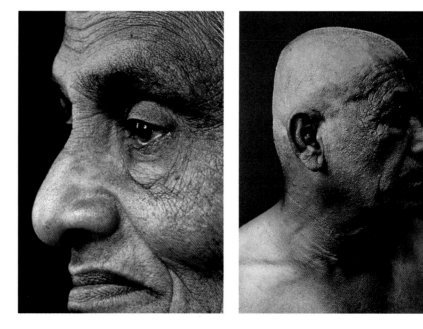

Daily routine exposure to the sun – even in very small doses and in more cloudy climates – can lead to long-term effects that increase our apparent age.

The part of the sunlight that causes most damage to the skin is called **ultraviolet radiation** (UVR), mentioned on page 39. Scientists have identified three kinds of UVR, called A, B and C radiation.

Some exposure to ultraviolet B is necessary, since it is essential for vitamin D production in the skin. The amount required is tiny, however, and 15 minutes a day is probably sufficient even in cloudy countries. Occasional exposure to visible sunlight is believed to enhance psychological well-being. The treatment of skin disorders such as psoriasis has in the past relied on deliberate controlled exposure to sunlight and to UVA lamps, but modern medicine offers alternatives today.

In spite of these benefits, however, the UV radiation from the sun is the environmental factor that is overall most damaging to the skin. People who have not been over-exposed to the sun for many years will tend to have pale and unmarked skin; even those with significant pigment will look paler than their kin. Sun worshippers will look very different.

Sun tanning and sunburn

Sun **tanning** is a response to the damaging effects of ultraviolet radiation. In people with pale skins sunlight stimulates the melanocytes to increase melanin pigment production, and also increases the transfer of melanosomes to keratinocytes. This melanocyte response to sunlight results in tanning, and by dramatically increasing melanin production provide an immediate and important defence for the nuclei of the skin cells.

In people with dark skins the much higher levels of melanin offer inherent protection by up to 30 times that of type I skins, though they do not offer complete protection.

Initially, acutely sun-damaged skin develops a thickened epidermis. This is caused by faster cell renewal, which is part of the immediate defence mechanism of the skin. The epidermis will return to normal provided the skin is not repeatedly over-exposed.

As everyone knows, acute over-exposure to the sun results in **sunburn**. Intense redness is produced by increased blood flow due to the release of chemicals by damaged cells.

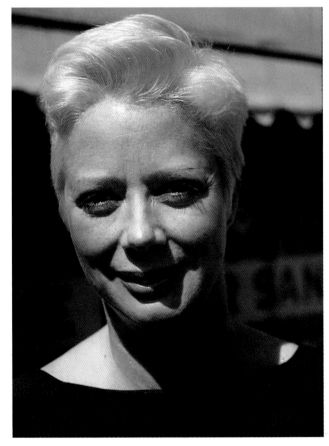

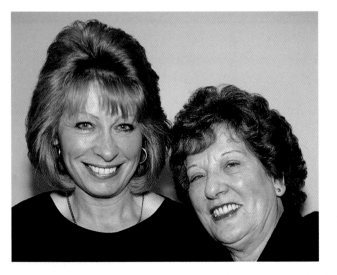

People who have not been regularly exposed to the sun tend to have light and unmarked skin; a habitual sun worshipper shows a strong and persistent response to UVR.

THE TYPES OF ULTRAVIOLET RADIATION

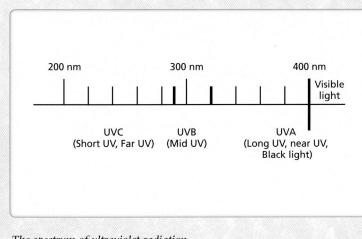

The spectrum of ultraviolet radiation.

- **Ultraviolet C** (UVC, 100–280 nm) is the most energetic of all UVR, and the most dangerous in terms of the damage it can inflict on living material. This has not greatly affected humans until now; having been mostly removed within the atmosphere, mainly by absorption in the ozone layer, it did not reach the earth's surface in any harmful quantity. The well-publicised 'thinning' of the ozone layer that has taken place in the last few decades has increased the amounts that reach our planet, however, especially in the Southern Hemisphere.

- **Ultraviolet B** (UVB, 280–315nm) is the most damaging part of UVR that we encounter. It is currently thought to generate most of the photodamage to skin, though not all. UVB is mostly blocked by dense clouds, closely woven clothing and glass window panes. Significant amounts are transmitted from blue sky in the middle of the day in summer. It is less dangerous when the sun is low in the sky, at high latitude in winter, and in early mornings and late evenings in summer.

- **Ultraviolet A** (UVA, 315–400nm) is about 1000 times less damaging to the skin than UVB. On the other hand, 20 times more UVA than UVB reaches the earth in the middle of a summer's day. It is not greatly affected by absorption and scattering in the atmosphere when the sun is low in the sky, and is now known to contribute significantly to the total exposure at moderate levels throughout the whole day and year. UVA penetrates deeper into the skin and leads to deeper damage than UVB does. It penetrates cloud cover, light clothing and untinted glass relatively easily, and may induce a degree of continuing skin damage over long periods, even when UVR exposure is not obvious.

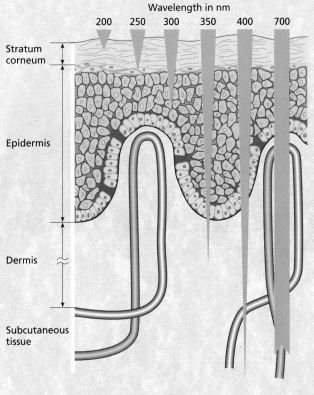

The depth of penetration of the skin by UV radiation of different wavelengths: UVB mainly affects the epidermis, while UVA penetrates deeper into the dermis.

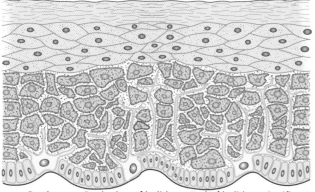

Resting   Beginning of holidays   End of holidays: significant
melanocyte   melanocyte response

How skin pigmentation (represented by green coloration) develops during a holiday in a sun resort.

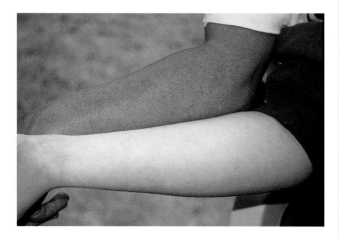

Sun tan is a defence against the sun. These two forearms reflect the difference in daily exposure to the sun over two weeks.

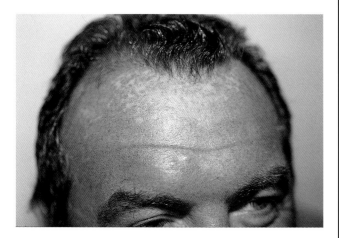

Severe sunburn, the result of acute and excessive exposure to the sun.

The epidermis, particularly the stratum corneum, is not able to control water effectively. Fortunately this can be rapidly remedied, especially if a good-quality moisturiser is used and further exposure avoided.

SUNBURN TREATMENT

- Take aspirin or paracetamol as soon as you detect any sunburn. Either of these drugs will help to reduce inflammation and control pain.
- Cool, wet compresses or cool soaks for 20 minutes four or five times daily will also help with pain control.
- Do not put butter or heavy ointments on the burned skin, as they can cause skin irritation.
- Increased fluid loss can occur through badly sunburned skin, so fluid replenishment with an 'isotonic' drink is recommended.
- Avoid more sun exposure until the skin completely heals, usually within one or two weeks. This is because sun-damaged skin is more susceptible to subsequent burns.

Constant exposure to sunlight causes the melanocytes to become chronically over-active, resulting in areas of excessive melanin in the skin. These form brown spots called **freckles**.

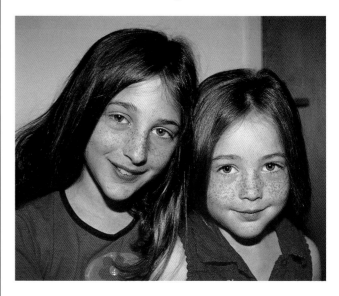

Overproduction of melanin in localised areas causes freckles.

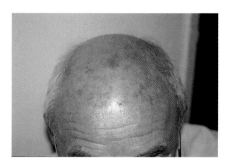

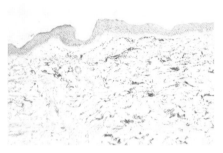

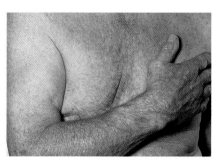

Solar lentigines, patches of pigmented skin. This gentleman has spent most of his life in the sun.

A section through badly sun-damaged skin. In skin like this the epidermis thickens and the skin may become leathery.

Photodamaged skin on the forearm.

Eventually, areas of damaged skin made up of increased numbers of melanocytes and increased melanin synthesis develop. These are called **solar lentigines**, and are the result of a lifetime of sun exposure.

Photodamage

Photoageing (which can make up to around 85% of the overall appearance of ageing) is a slow process. It proceeds for several decades before it becomes obvious. The degree of photoageing is determined by the skin type and by the *total* lifetime sun exposure. People who spend their lives almost entirely indoors show very little sun-induced skin damage.

Moreover, the degree of damage to tissues in different regions of the body is directly proportional to the amount of sunlight received. Everyone is familiar, for example, with the sharp boundary between exposed and unexposed skin that often develops in the V-area of the neck.

In chronically sun-damaged skin the epidermis as a whole becomes thicker, and loses some of its undulations. In young people the thickness of the epidermis is between 35 and 50 micrometres. At the age of 70 in skin that has been protected it could be expected to be between 25 and 40 micrometres. In sun-damaged skin it may be much more than this.

This is probably because marginally more daughter cells are produced by the basal layer, and produced more quickly. The effect is that the spiny layer and the granular layer thicken up. The stratum corneum, on the other hand, does not change very much, except that the cells within it (the corneocytes) increase still more in surface area and may become even thinner. The speed at which cells are replaced slows down, and some of the functions of skin, including controlling water loss, may become less efficient. There is less elasticity and increased fragility. Skin becomes dry, flaky and less reflective of light.

As photoageing begins, the small blood capillaries in the dermis decrease in number and the remaining blood vessels become tortuous and dilated. The elastic fibres degenerate, in a process called **elastosis**, producing a thickened mass that replaces the collagen.

A steady accumulation of damaged elastic fibres is accompanied by deterioration of the surrounding tissues until a blue-grey tangle of swollen, degenerate fibres, quite unlike normal skin, develops in the upper part of the dermis.

These changes in the elastic fibres are not seen in skin that has always been protected, even in very old people. Curiously enough, the changes can be quite advanced before the extent of the damage becomes visible.

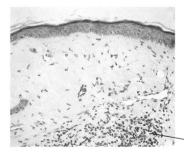

Section through skin taken from the arm (a 'biopsy'), showing the long-term results of collagen and elastin disorganisation – elastosis and chronic thickening of the epidermis.

Elastosis

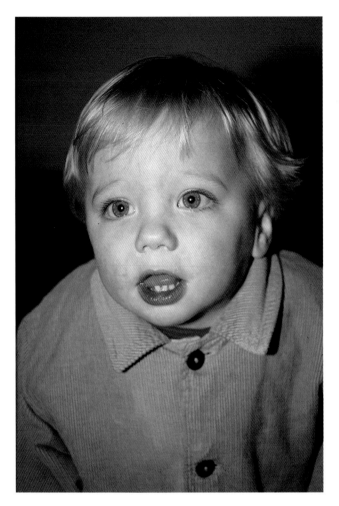

It is all-important that the skin of young children should be protected from the sun: parents' care at this stage can help to avoid disease and disfigurement in later life.

Seriously photoaged skin is dry, deeply wrinkled, yellow and rough. It may be marked with darkly pigmented or whitish spots, which respectively show where levels of pigment are higher or lower than normal. With increasing sun damage small blood vessels in the dermis will become more obvious and will form the red, finely branching, spider-like marks ('broken veins') that doctors call **telangiectases**. These blood vessels are easily damaged, resulting in greater fragility of the skin, with the development of spots called **purpura**.

Loss of elastic fibres around the blood vessels of the lower lips and ears – areas especially sensitive to chronic sun damage – may result in dilated veins. On the other hand, in protected skin the vessels tend not to be so dilated or damaged.

At its worst, skin that has been over-exposed to the sun for many years looks like old leather. Moreover, constant exposure to UVR over many years can result in warty spots on the skin, called **actinic keratoses**.

These are found most often in people with type I and type II skins, although even people with type VI skins can develop them, and then only on the areas of the skin exposed to the sun. The appearance of actinic keratoses means that the skin has received far too much sun and could develop a **skin cancer** eventually.

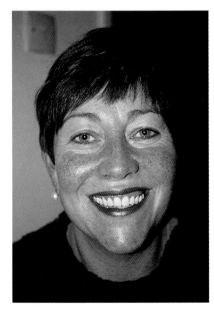

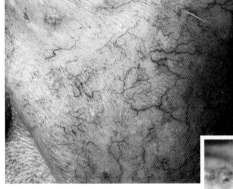

Telangiectases and purpura – fine, branching, red spider-like marks and spots – develop on sun-exposed skin.

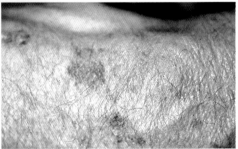

Purpura are spots due to sun-damaged blood vessels

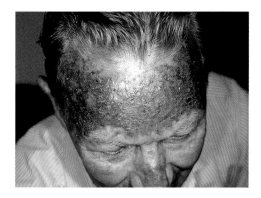

Actinic keratoses are defects in the skin due to chronic photodamage.

The common skin cancers are most often seen in older people. **Basal cell carcinomas**, are seen on the face, especially in the area around the eyes and the nose. They are the commonest of all cancers in humans. **Squamous cell carcinomas** are more aggressive and invasive. They usually occur on the back of the hands, on the ears or on the edges of lips.

Actinic keratoses and basal and squamous cell carcinomas occur mainly on exposed areas of the skin, and are the result of excessive sun exposure over many years, often commencing in childhood: we receive 80% of our total sun exposure before we reach the age of 18.

Melanomas are the best known type of skin cancer. They are increasingly recognised by the public as a potential health hazard, especially if a mole changes shape or colour or begins to bleed, when they may become what is called a malignant melanoma.

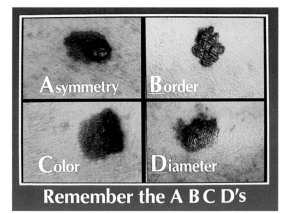

Look out for these four changes in a deeply pigmented mole:
Asymmetry – has it become more irregular in shape?
Border – has it increased rapidly?
Colour – has it darkened noticeably?
Diameter – has it increased in size?

If you have a skin mark like this, and notice changes in it, see your doctor immediately.

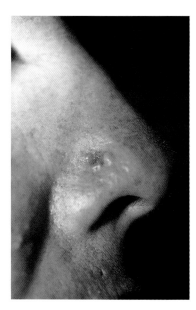

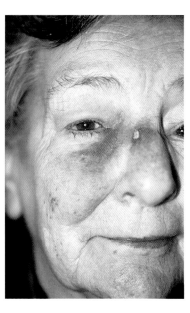

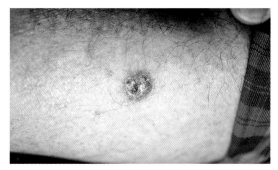

▲ Squamous cell carcinomas: these are aggressive cancers and can spread.

◄ Basal cell carcinomas on the face and scalp are the commonest human cancer. They are caused by sun exposure, often commencing in childhood. This type of cancer would develop in almost all of us if UVR levels were to increase substantially.

Photoprotective products

Ultraviolet radiation can seriously damage exposed skin of all skin types. As we have seen, as well as aesthetic damage linked to premature skin ageing, it also carries the risk of skin cancer. The problem is made worse by the fashion for sunbathing in summer in certain cultures. In winter, skiing can also lead to high UV exposure.

Photoprotection – protection of the skin from UVR – has an important role for all skins. The ideal protection product would incorporate the following:

- effective absorption of radiation (both UVB and UVA)
- resistance to water and sweat
- stability in daylight and in air, and also to heat
- total safety for the skin.

The ability of a product to absorb radiation are defined by its **sun protection factor** (SPF). Scientists measure the SPF of a product by measuring the time it takes to develop slight skin redness (**erythema**) to a known amount of radiation. This time is termed the **minimum erythema dose** (MED). The MED for a product containing sunscreen can be measured against one without, on the same area of skin. Suppose, for example, that:

MED with photoprotector = 300 minutes

and

MED without photoprotector = 10 minutes

then

the SPF of this product = 300/10 = 30.

An SPF of, say, 30 is no guarantee, however, that one can stay in the sun 30 times longer than when not wearing a sunscreen. This is because the product may be altered – for instance, if the wearer goes for a swim or rubs the product off!

Sunscreens

The regular, daily use of modern cosmetic products can potentially be very important for the long-term health of the skin. Among the most useful ingredients are **sunscreens**, which block ultraviolet radiation absorption by the skin, either wholly or in part. (Clothing, hats and sunglasses can all act as effective sunscreens.) The many formulations that are on sale include lotions, creams, pastes and gels, and rely on either chemical or physical agents for their protective action.

Packaging should indicate (left) the protection offered by a product against both UVA and UVB radiation, and also (right) the degree of protection.

/e skin the moisturisation and)k its best now and in the future.

nique balance
)rotection
l complex.

on is
matologists.

D A I L Y
UVA/B
PROTECTION LEVEL
RECOMMENDED BY
DERMATOLOGISTS

OLOGICALLY TESTED & PROVEN
LY COMBINATION SKIN

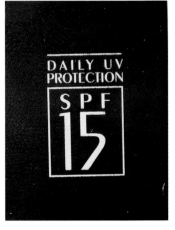

DAILY UV
PROTECTION

S P F
15

SUN PROTECTION: SOME GUIDELINES

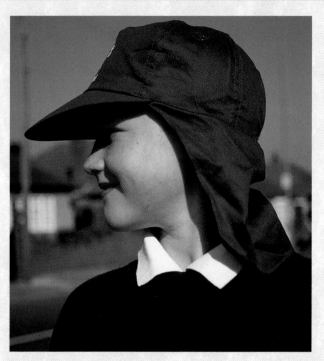

Really thorough sun protection!

- Sun damage is cumulative. All the doses of ultraviolet radiation (UVR) received by the skin, large or small, add up: the total dose leads to skin wrinkling, altered pigmentation and skin cancer. **Protect the children**!

- There is no such thing as a 'healthy tan'. Tanning is a response to skin injury by UVR.

- Avoid sun exposure between the hours of 11 a.m. to 2 p.m., when UVB is most intense. Plan outdoor activities for the early morning or late afternoon.

- Protect the skin with clothing first, and apply sunscreen to any remaining unprotected skin. Wear a hat!

- Apply sunscreens **even on overcast days**. Although UVR is less intense on overcast days, UVA is still present and adds to the cumulative skin damage.

- Beware of sun exposure at high altitudes. In the mountains there is less atmosphere to absorb UVR, and therefore the risk of sunburn is greater.

- UVR is strongest near the equator, where the sun's rays strike the earth most directly.

- UVR is reflected by sand, concrete and snow, and reflected UVR adds to the total exposure. Because UVR is reflected and scattered, sitting in the shade does not necessarily protect from sunburn.

- Although sun beds emit mostly UVA, over-exposure can still cause sunburn, and their use enhances skin ageing and the risk of skin cancer. Beauty therapists will counsel their clients accordingly.

- People at high risk for skin cancer (persons with skin types I and II, outdoor workers, and persons with a history of skin cancer or a photosensitivity) should use sunscreens daily, and should never 'sunbathe'.

- Keep babies out of the sun. Begin using sunscreens on children as soon as they learn to walk, and then allow sun exposure with moderation.

- Teach children sun protection early.

- Use a good-quality skin care product, such as a moisturiser containing sunscreen ingredients with an SPF factor (see page 78) of at least 15, and active against UVA and UVB. Use it regularly, *every* day.

Chemical sunscreens are synthetic chemical substances with the following properties:

- they are powerful absorbers of UV radiation
- when they absorb radiation they remain relatively stable, and release the absorbed energy quite slowly.

These sun filters are formulated with other compounds in order to obtain highly effective products with protection factors varying from 2 to 30. As with all products applied to the skin, however, some of the ingredients may be absorbed through the skin (**percutaneous absorption**), which may cause some irritation in a few people. Moreover, they often have to be reapplied quite frequently.

For many people, however, the advantages of chemical sunscreens outweigh the disadvantages. With all products it is advisable to read the label, to check that the product blocks both UVB and UVA radiation.

Physical sunscreens contain inert mineral particles that reflect UV rays like a mirror. The most common type used is ultrafine titanium dioxide (TiO_2), made up of minute particles only 20–30 nm^3 in size.

These products have advantages over chemical sunscreens in that they are inert substances that do not break down over time. They are far less liable to cause skin irritation, since they are in the form of insoluble particles that are not absorbed through the skin. Because of the small size of the particles, modern physical sunscreens reflect radiation in the UVB and short UVA regions better than earlier products did. Also, whereas their predecessors left a slight residue on the skin that looked like a trace of make-up base, which some people found unattractive, today's products have better transparency and avoid this problem.

There are formulations for use on the face and lips, and special preparations that can be used by small children. All should be reapplied after sweating or swimming, even if the product claims to be waterproof and rub-proof, or to offer 'all-day protection'. Ideally, whichever sunscreen you choose, make sure that it blocks both UVB and UVA and has a sun protection factor (SPF) rating of at least 15. Only the brave, or the foolhardy, will risk a lower rating than this!

Slip, slap, slop

In Australia the Government and doctors led a public information program to reduce the effects of sun damage. They used the slogan 'Slip, slap, slop':

Slip on a tee-shirt, slap on a hat and slop on some sun cream.

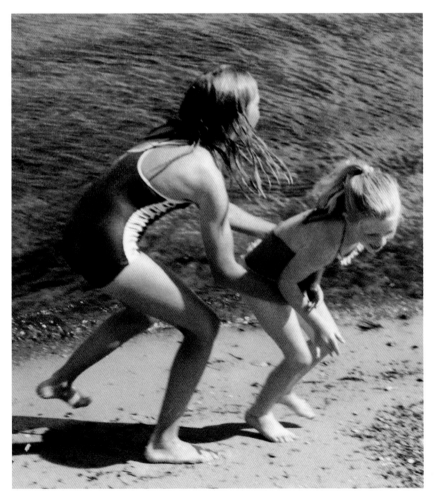

Children experience massive UV exposure. Protection against UVA and UVB is the only way to be sure of preventing long-term damage.

Self-tanning products

Over the last twenty years or so, people have developed a growing awareness of the harmful effects of sun on the skin. Nevertheless many people would still like to look tanned. Out of this contradiction arose the category of **self-tanning products**. These are preparations that induce a skin coloration similar to the colour resulting from exposure of the skin to UV light.

All such products on the market today contain **dihydroxyacetone** (DHA) as the active ingredient that produces the brown coloration of the skin. (Others, such as glyceraldehyde, 6-aldo-D-fructose, erythrulose and glucose, have been shown to induce skin coloration to a lesser extent.) Modern products have overcome the unpleasant smell and feel of the older ones.

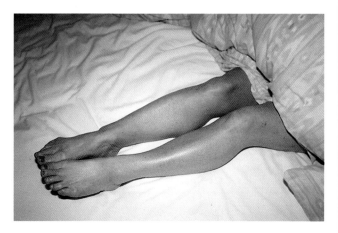

A self-tanning product has been used here on one leg only, to illustrate its effectiveness. It provides a safe way of attaining the desired aesthetic effect of a sun-tan.

Through a series of reactions, DHA reacts with the skin's amino acids to create the brown-coloured product that makes the skin look naturally tanned. This reaction is not immediate, and usually takes from two to three hours for the full development of colour on the skin. Once the coloration has developed, it will remain and will resist washing, since it is part of the skin cells' amino acid structure. It does not provide any protection from UV light, however, and cannot be considered as a sunscreen.

The colour gradually fades as the cells themselves are lost through the natural desquamation process. Depending on the number of stratum corneum cell layers that are coloured through the reaction with DHA, it usually takes five or six days for the colour to disappear completely.

Modern self-tanning products continue a high proportion of silicones, which improve their spreadability and thereby reduce the risk of streaking.

The use of self-tanning products is a reasonable alternative for the health-conscious consumer who is determined to look tanned but who has finally understood that lengthy exposure to the sun will result at best in the acceleration of the ageing process, and at worst in skin cancer.

Reducing lines and wrinkles

People who have noticed the effects of skin ageing and sun damage often try to improve their appearance, and using specialist products can help. Cleansers and moisturisers containing ingredients called **hydroxy acids** enhance the process of renewing the stratum corneum by reducing the strength of the bonds between its cells. Cleopatra is said to have bathed in asses' milk, which contains an alpha-hydroxy acid, to clear her skin.

Alpha-hydroxy acids, often called 'fruit acids', are used in many cosmetic products to speed up cell renewal; lactic and glycolic acids are widely used. Recently a **beta-hydroxy acid** called salicylic acid has been shown to aid the

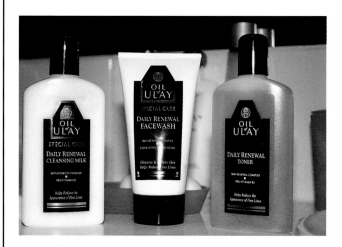

Specialist products containing beta-hydroxy acids.

desquamation process without significantly reducing the water content of the stratum corneum or increasing TEWL, which may result in skin irritation. The beta-hydroxy acids do not penetrate deeply into the epidermis. The regular use of products containing hydroxy acids can make fine lines appear less obvious by enhancing hydration and desquamation.

Exfoliation carried out by a beauty therapist has a similar effect. (See Chapter 7, 'At the beauty salon'.)

More dramatic results can be achieved by chemical **facial peels**, which contain very high levels of hydroxy acids such as glycolic acid, or even phenol. In some countries women choose to have these done regularly. Facial peels should only be carried out by experienced practitioners, however, as they can lead to scarring.

Laser surgery is also employed for this purpose, and the results can be strikingly effective. If it is performed inexpertly, however, the side-effects can be devastating.

SKIN REJUVENATION: TRUTH OR MYTH?

There are no known therapies or products that can rejuvenate aged skin. There are medical and cosmetic products that make the skin *appear* younger, however.

In scientific studies some cosmetic products have been shown to make fine lines less noticeable by improving skin hydration.

A few substances, of which isotretinoin is an example, have been found to improve the effects of sun damage to some degree. At the time of writing, however, these may only be prescribed by doctors, and it is not certain whether the amounts permitted in cosmetic products have any beneficial effect.

INCI name	Function
Aqua (water)	Solvent
PPG-15 stearyl ester	Salicylic acid solubiliser
Glycerin	Skin conditioning agent/humectant
Stearyl alcohol	Thickener/stabiliser
Salicylic acid	Exfoliant
Cetyl betaine	Surfactant/cleansing agent
Distearyldimonium chloride	Thickener
Sodium lauryl sulfate	Surfactant/cleansing agent
Oxidised polyethylene	Exfoliant agent
Parfum	Fragrance
Cetyl alcohol	Thickener/stabiliser
Behenyl alcohol	Thickener/stabiliser
Steareth-21	Emulsifier
Steareth-2	Emulsifier
PPG-30	Salicylic acid stabiliser
Disodium EDTA	Chelator
BHT	Preservative

The ingredients of a high-quality modern cleanser containing salicylic acid (a beta-hydroxy acid, an aid to desquamation), and their functions.

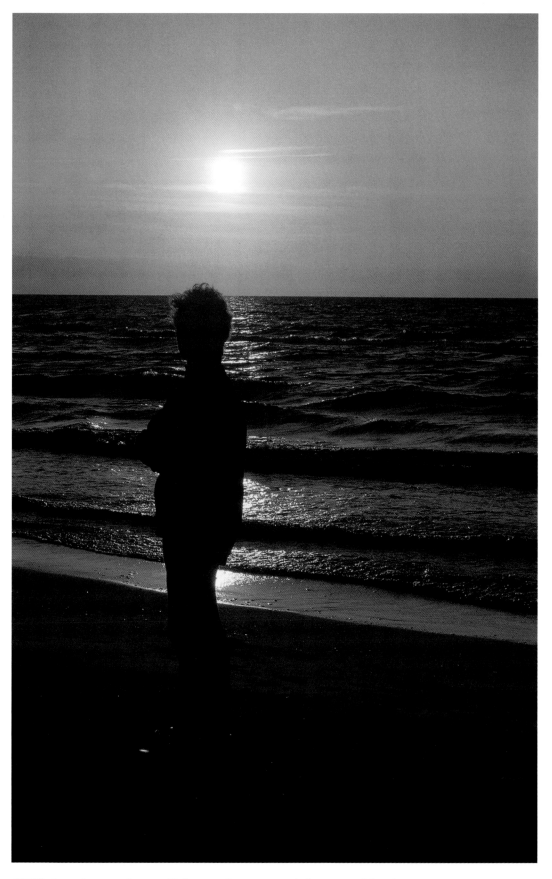

All life depends upon the sun. Unfortunately, some people have a terrible price to pay.

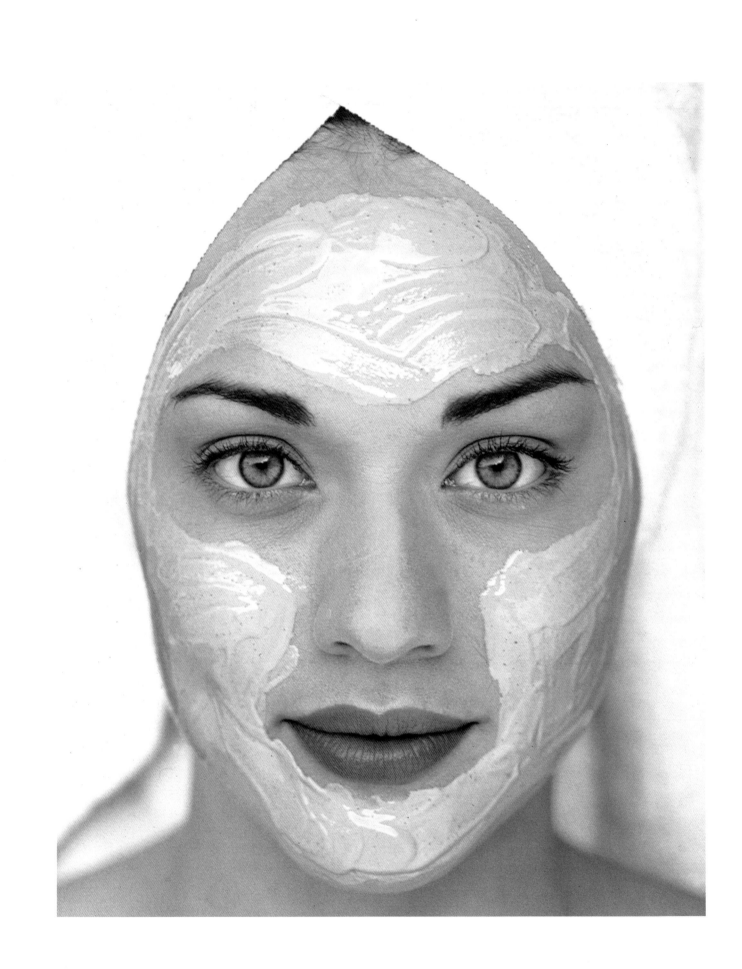

5
Skin care

Looking after the skin means different things to different people. To some it means nothing more than a splosh with water or a scrub with a soap bar, carried out as thoroughly, regularly and frequently as the other claims made on one's time permit.

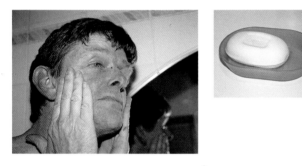

A quick splash with soap and water is the only skin care routine for many people, particularly men...

To others it means a regular skin care routine of cleansing, toning and moisturising, involving considerable expenditure of time and the use of

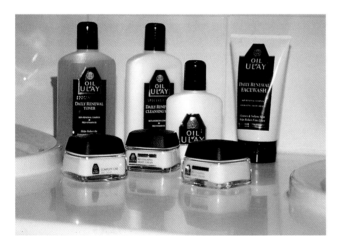

... whereas others employ cleansing, toning and moisturising; the more 'sophisticated' the society, the more products seem to be used.

many cosmetic products, sometimes several times a day, often followed by the application of decorative cosmetics.

The cosmetic industry (and its customers) have to face up to its critics, including some doctors, who accuse it of the excessive promotion of cosmetic products that they consider to be irrelevant to skin care.

But how many of us understand how our skin benefits by cleansing and moisturising to combat the effects of constant immersion and the daily damage done by the environment and the wearing of decorative cosmetics? Most people need information on skin function, as well as advice on to how to meet their skin's specific needs.

From the day we are born our skin, though astonishingly robust and renewable, needs some care. Skin care involves both protection and treatment: protection against the long-term effects of the sun, wind and water, together with management of whatever happens to the skin on a day-to-day basis.

It is never too early to start looking after your skin, or that of your child.

In this chapter we talk about skin care from birth to old age. We look at the types of product available, and examine how they work.

Diet, vitamins and the skin

Week by week, magazine articles carry dozens of suggestions as to how we could make our skin healthier, including some that are startlingly improbable. In addition, recommendations for special and exotic diets, and hosts of vitamin supplements, are constantly being offered to those who are interested in improving their skin.

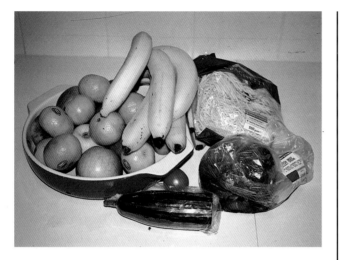

A varied well-balanced diet includes plenty of fruit and vegetables; most healthy people don't need extra vitamin supplements.

SKIN MYTH

Generous doses of vitamin supplements are vital to healthy skin.

Fact: It is true that a well-balanced diet is essential for our general health. Vitamin A prevents skin from becoming dry and flaky, vitamin C is important for the production of collagen and vitamin E helps to rehydrate the skin, damp down inflammation and speed up the healing process.

Only tiny amounts of vitamins are necessary for health, however, and these amounts are easily found in any good, varied diet. It can be positively harmful to take more than these amounts.

In fact it takes very considerable dietary deficiencies to harm the skin. Swallowing vast amounts of supplements – and some people unwisely take them in doses far in excess of those recommended on the pack – cannot make the skin look healthier. Think, for example, how the clearest and healthiest skins are those of children before puberty, even though many of them live on what their parents feel is 'junk food'.

As we have seen, healthy skin is the consequence of a well-hydrated and intact epidermis, together with avoidance of sun damage.

Smoking and your skin

It is wise to avoid smoking, if for no other reason than that it damages the appearance of the skin. (There are other, even better, reasons too!) Cigarette smoke and tar deprive the skin of the nutrients and oxygen it needs for good health, ultimately leaving it looking dull and lifeless. They lead to the formation of harmful free radicals and weaken the collagen and elastin fibres, with the result that the skin becomes prematurely wrinkled.

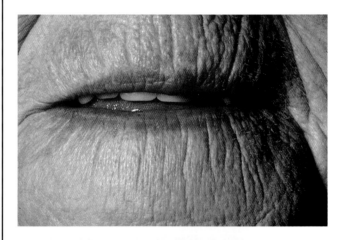

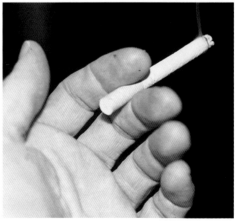

Smoking damages the skin, and may also cause secondary wrinkling as the face – particularly the lips – responds to the smoke.

Skin care throughout life

Infant skin

Every new parent takes a great delight and a tender satisfaction in looking at, and touching, the delicate skin of a newborn baby. It is a lifelong challenge to maintain this delicate skin.

Some newborn babies, especially those that have arrived prematurely, have very little subcutaneous fat, with the result that their skin lies loosely over their muscles and bones. As a result they have a somewhat wrinkly start. The skin of a premature baby can comprise up to 13% of its body weight, compared with 3% in an adult.

The skin of a full-term infant has a well-developed epidermis, similar to that of an adult. A premature baby, however, has fewer layers of stratum corneum. This results in increased permeability and increased TEWL, and is one of the reasons why very premature babies are so vulnerable. But by the age of 10–14 days, the skin of even the youngest premature babies has begun to function as a reasonable barrier to fluid and heat losses, and is less permeable to substances applied to its surface.

Another variation in the skin structure and function involves the connection of the epidermis to the dermis. At this junction there are normally numerous anchoring rete pegs (see page 10), but in the skin of premature babies these are fewer and more widely spread. Premature babies are therefore more vulnerable to blistering, and care is needed when removing adhesives to avoid stripping off the epidermis.

Soaps that are used for routine bathing include 'baby soaps', soaps formulated to have a neutral pH, superfatted soaps and even deodorant soaps with antimicrobial properties. All soaps are, at best, mild irritants to the skin, and frequent soaping increases the irritant effect. Specially formulated synthetic cleansing products called syndets are preferable to soaps (see page 98).

Moisturisers

Lubricants such as creams, emollients and 'baby lotions' or oils may be used for newborn babies, whether premature or not, to prevent or treat dryness of the skin as it meets a more hostile environment.

Diaper dermatitis

Wet areas of skin that are kept covered may be prone to damage. Nappy rash (diaper dermatitis) is seldom the result of the inadequate washing

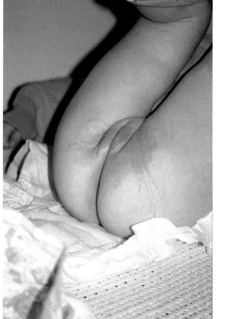
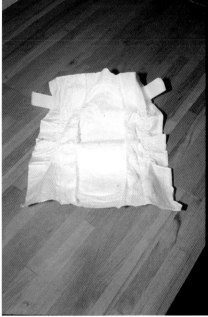

Soreness in the nappy region (diaper dermatitis) can make babies uncomfortable and fretful, but paper diapers have helped to greatly reduce the incidence of this condition over the last 20 years.

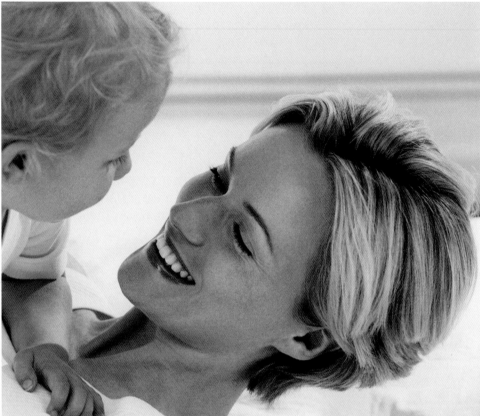

A baby's skin plays an essential part in the bonding of a mother and her young child.

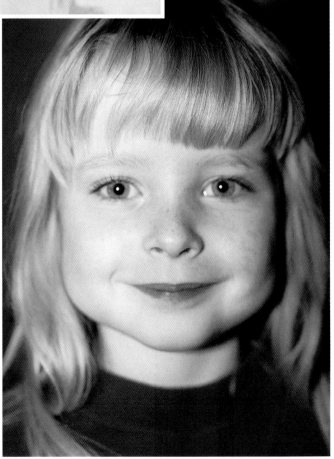

The beautiful undamaged skin of childhood: perhaps the healthiest we are likely to see.

of nappies, though it may follow their inadequate drying, or inadequate washing or constant wetness of the skin. Today's technologically advanced paper diapers, which hold urine and faeces away from the skin, have helped to reduce the frequency of this condition significantly over the last 20 years.

It is far better and easier to prevent nappy rash than to have to treat it. Methods of prevention include keeping the skin dry with frequent nappy changes, or the use of highly absorbent nappies that pull moisture away from the skin so that it is not softened by being damp for long periods.

Barrier products that also remove harmful skin bacteria are helpful in reducing diaper dermatitis.

Childhood skin

After the early months of babyhood have passed the skin of most children has a more than adequate layer of fatty 'padding' which gives it a beautiful smooth appearance, often described as having the quality of 'purity'. All the functions are very active, and because the stratum corneum is functioning effectively the skin is very well hydrated. Indeed, by and large children's skin is the healthiest we ever see.

A child's skin shows little or no damage from sunlight. Children have more leisure time than they will ever enjoy again, however, and many of them play outside whenever they can, often spending most of the summer out of doors. There is often massive exposure to the sun during childhood, which will have long-term consequences.

The care of the skin of small children is almost entirely in the hands of parents or other carers. Nevertheless it is never too soon for them to begin to learn about skin care. The skin does not need moisturising unless there is atopy or eczema, or after prolonged exposure to sun or sea, but regular protection against the sun should begin *now*.

It is vital to protect the skin of children against the sun, and particularly against sunburn, to prevent the development of skin cancer in the years ahead.

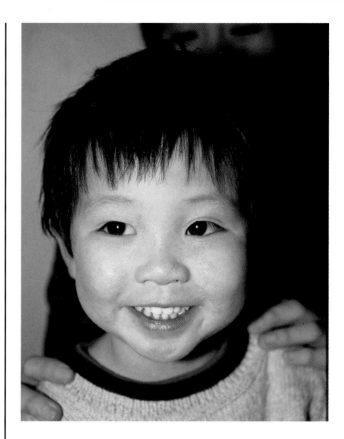

Adolescence

As we reach our teens that lovely smooth skin of childhood undergoes some terrifying changes – just as we get interested in the other sex.

As we have seen, this is the time of life at which the body starts to produce greatly increased amounts of sex hormones. Both girls and boys produce male hormones, called **androgens**. Under the influence of these androgens the skin produces more grease (sebum) and in most teenagers there is a tendency for spots to develop. These can be anything from simple blackheads to large pustules.

Caring for teenage skin is a matter of balancing the cleansing and toning needed to remove the excess grease with adequate moisturising to combat the potential over-drying effects of this cleaning. Young people's skins tend to hold water well, so they need far lighter moisturisers than those formulated for elderly people, whose skin tends naturally to be dry. Even at this age, cleansing and moisturising products should contain ingredients that screen against UVA and UVB.

Young skin regime: meticulous cleansing and moisturising, part of the necessary care for a truly sensitive (atopic) skin.

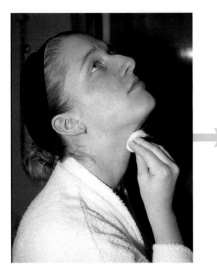 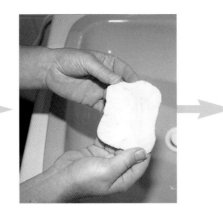 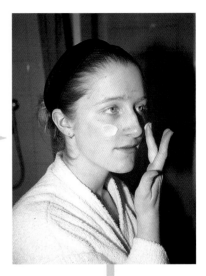

First remove dead squames and detritus using a mild synthetic cleanser on a cotton pad…

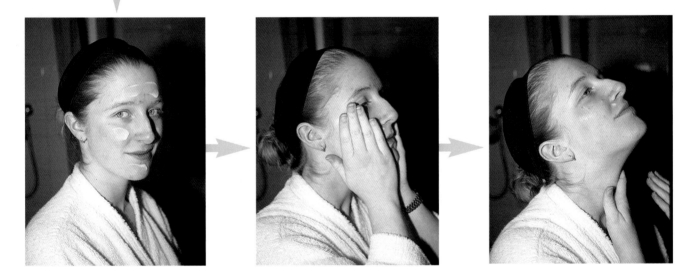

… then apply moisturiser to face and throat, using the fingertips to ensure even distribution.

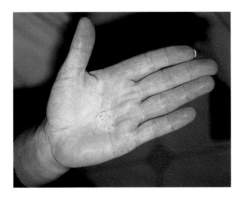

The right amount of moisturiser to use.

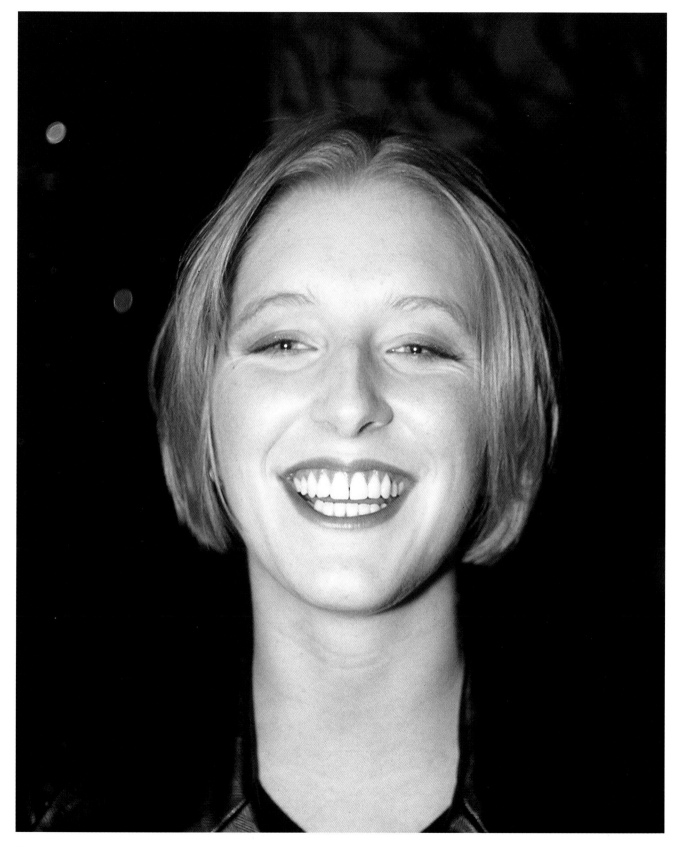

Young women have to cope not only with the complexities of greasy skin but with an increasing use of decorative cosmetics (lipsticks, eye shadow and liner) and their removal, all of which need to be taken into account when deciding on a skin care routine.

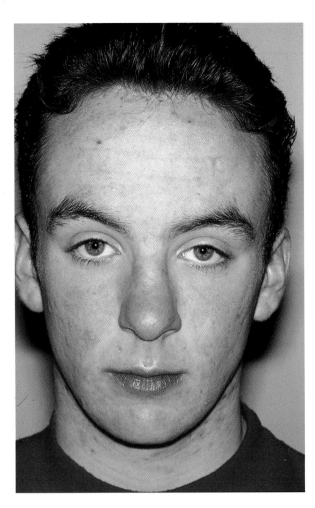

In adolescence, increasing sebum secretion under the influence of the rising levels of male hormones leads to a greasy skin. The condition usually clears with the arrival of adulthood.

Adult skin

Whatever our nationality or race, our skin changes inexorably as we get older.

A young adult's skin is well hydrated, tends to be soft, smooth and supple, and has a natural translucency; by contrast, in the natural course of things a more mature adult skin tends to function less well. Ultimately it may become dry and tend to feel tight, with a rougher texture and duller appearance, and wrinkles start to appear.

Wrinkles are the result of a combination of factors:

- a gradual reduction in the water content of the stratum corneum, lipids and sebum
- some degree of photodamage.

This gradual deterioration in skin appearance and function is what drives many people to seek skin care products that reduce the appearance of lines and at the same time are effective moisturisers against the increasing dryness. (Surveys show that most mature women are concerned more with the discomfort of dryness than with visible wrinkles.) The ability to procure such products and use them regularly is dependent on income and availability, which varies widely worldwide.

Cleansing may become less frequent as the excessive sebum production of adolescence declines, but the use of a heavier-duty night moisturiser without sunscreens should be added to the skin care routine. Ingredients that modify the appearance of fine lines are now incorporated into some high-quality cosmetic products. Exfoliation (see page 109) improves the 'feel' of skin, but should be regarded with caution by people who have sensitive skins: it may be used once or twice a week, depending on the skin type, need and the mildness of the product. The regular use of heavier-duty moisturisers for the hands is helpful, and indeed is essential for people in 'wet work' such as cleaners, hairdressers and cement workers.

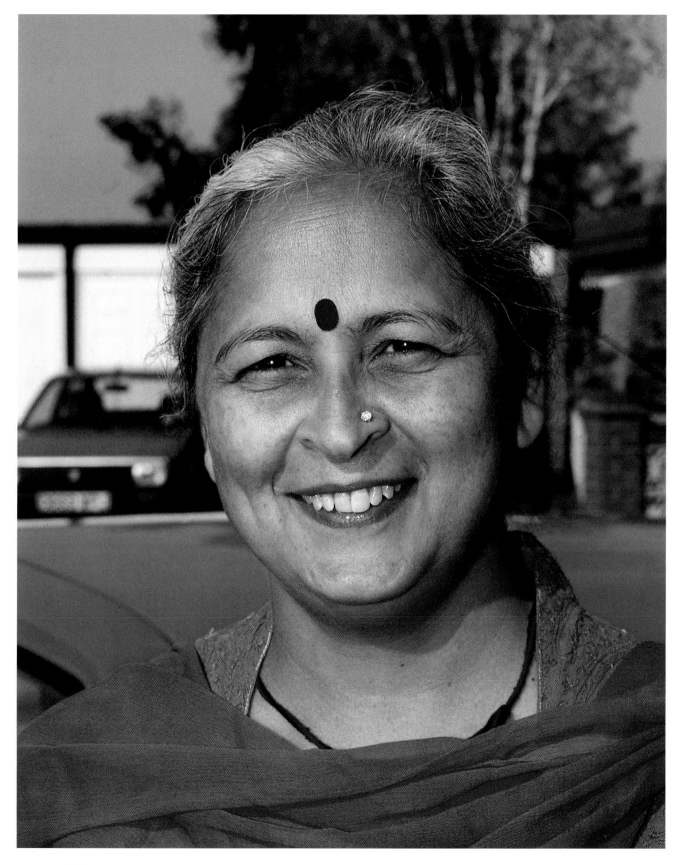

Women of all races use decorative cosmetics: here the traditional bindhi, worn by many Indian women on the forehead. Removing cosmetics is an important part of skin care, often forgotten by those who criticise the use of cleansers and moisturisers.

In developing countries women may have to resort to local and 'natural' products. 'Natural' does not necessarily mean 'better', however, or even 'safe'. Natural products made from vegetable or animal extracts may be inherently toxic, and if prepared locally the concentrations of active ingredients cannot be controlled.

The cosmetic industry uses only ingredients that have established scientific profiles, and then only in legal and known concentrations. Many ingredients of skin care products have to be prepared synthetically, since their 'natural' counterparts are far more likely to be harmful.

Mature skin

As women get older and their skin matures, and particularly after the change of life (menopause), declining oestrogen may lead to dehydration of the stratum corneum, which tends to make the skin look thinner and older than it really is.

For cleansing, it may be advisable to use superfatted soaps or soap-free cleansers for the body. It is often preferable to use, say, a cleansing milk for the face.

It is essential to choose a suitable moisturising cream for use on the facial skin. If the cream is to give sufficient protection against

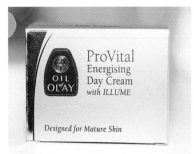

Skin care products specially formulated for mature skin, designed to improve moisturisation where the skin can be considerably compromised.

dehydration, it must have sufficient covering power to slow down the loss of water from the stratum corneum.

The use of a moisturising cream on the body skin can be useful, especially in winter when the skin tends to be drier. Modern shower products contain moisturisers as well as cleansers. It may be helpful too to use a bath oil, added to the water in the bath. It is however best to avoid long scalding soaks, as well as harsh soaps and bath foams if the skin is sensitive as this combination disrupts its barrier function.

Elderly skin

By the time we reach old age our skin may well have experienced decades of sun exposure, even if only at very low levels. This is associated with the effects of intrinsic ageing. The result as we see it is almost always a balance of the two.

Elderly skin can be very dry and almost paper-thin, with the structures in the dermis clearly visible. The TEWL is increased, and the skin becomes more fragile and prone to injuries: with the lack of protection from the dermis, the small blood vessels become vulnerable to breakage and bursting ('broken veins').

Regular care is now especially important, including the use of mild cleansers. Good-quality day and (especially) night moisturisers will help to combat the decline in the skin's barrier function. It is still important to continue protecting the skin against the sun, although most of the damage has been done by now.

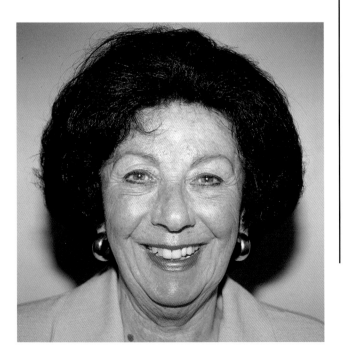

This lady takes great care of her skin, always using soap-free cleansers and a regular moisturiser formulated for mature skin.

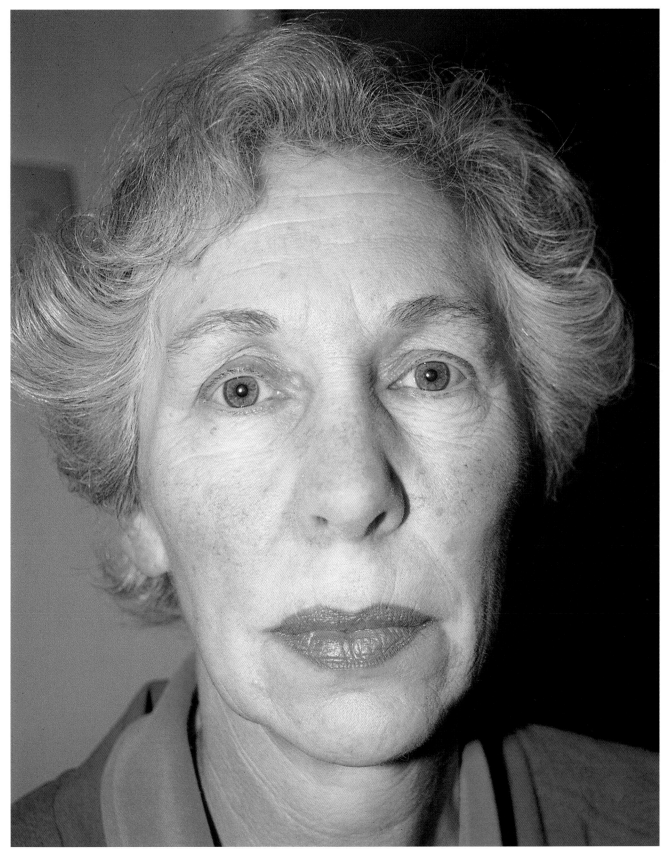

Elderly people may have skin like rice paper. All the dermal structure can be seen (although this lady takes exceptionally good care of her skin).

General guidelines for skin care

Whatever our nationality or race, our skin care habits have some similarities of objective, even if the degrees of sophistication of the products we use are very different.

In theory 'normal' skin does not need any modification, since it is already well balanced with respect to its physiological and mechanical integrity. Nevertheless, this balance can be unstable to some extent, and therefore two essential approaches to the care of normal skin must be considered:

- maintenance of this balance, and
- protection from external injury.

The first aim is a passive one: it is more particularly concerned with avoiding products that are not active treatments as such, but may be harmful to the skin – harsh soaps, for example. The second plays a more active role, involving the use of photoprotective products and hydrating agents.

Skin care, from the skin scientist's standpoint, means preserving the integrity of the stratum corneum while removing sebum and soiling and maintaining adequate moisturisation.

For most women throughout many centuries, this was achieved by very harsh and primitive means. Even until relatively recently, the only skin and hair care product used by most people was a bar of harsh soap.

Fortunately today's cosmetic industry is providing increasingly mild and sophisticated products at affordable prices which not only scientifically care for the skin, but also help to reduce the visible effects of ageing.

For most of us, skin care focuses on hands and face. Increasingly, however, industry is looking at the care of the body both in general and in specific areas, such as the delicate skin around the eyes, and good-quality products for these are now on the market.

In the rest of this chapter, we look at particular types of skin care and the products that are required for them.

Facial care

In this section we outline some suggestions for facial care regimens for skin of different ages.

Young (teenage) skin

Typical skin type – greasy /mixed:

- remove make-up
- cleanse, using mild products or a light cleanser such as a milk
- tone
- moisturise (using a light product, because of the presence of sebum, containing sunscreen ingredients that will block UVA/UVB.

Adult skin

Example skin type – normal to dry:

- remove make-up
- cleanse twice daily with a cleansing lotion or milk or with a mild bar soap (for men, this should include or be followed by a moisturiser)
- tone
- by day, use a medium moisturiser, with sunscreen ingredients (UVA/UVB)
- by night, use a heavier night cream without sunscreens
- moisturise hands regularly.

Elderly skin

Usual skin type – dry:

- cleanse with cream cleanser
- use heavy-duty moisturiser daily
- always use a night cream.

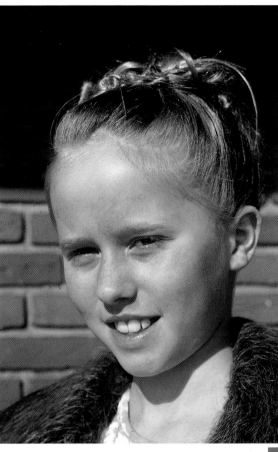

The skin of the face repays all the care we can give it, from childhood to maturity and beyond.

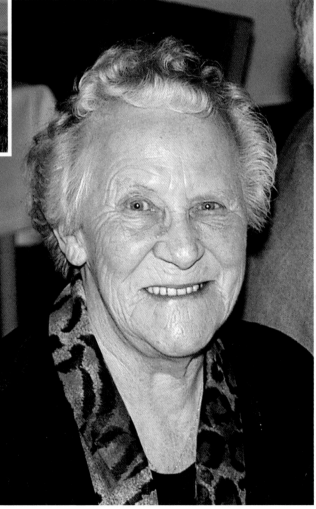

Skin cleansing

The aim of cleansing is to remove:

- surface dirt
- all make-up
- the top layer of dead skin cells
- potentially dangerous micro-organisms (bacteria).

The way in which any individual chooses to carry out this process is determined by habit, skin feel requirements and activity.

What goes to make a cleansing product?

For many generations **soaps** have been made by the extraction of oils and tallows from plants and animals and then treating these with alkalis to neutralise the fatty acids they contain. Soaps are good **emulsifiers** (that is, they hold solids in liquids in emulsion form so that they can be rinsed away), they have reasonable lathering power and an emollient action. Unfortunately, two problems are associated with soaps.

Firstly, because of their powerful cleansing action, overuse may completely eliminate the protective lipid film on the skin surface, which helps maintain the skin's physiological balance. As a result they may give rise to irritation.

Secondly, some soaps are alkaline (they have a high pH, around 9). Since skin pH is about 5, washing with soap leads to pH increases on the skin that can last for up to two hours. It has been suggested that this can lead to a growth of potentially harmful bacteria on the skin.

'Oily' soaps are enriched with **emollients** such as glycerol, fatty acids or oils, which have a softening and smoothing action. They can leave the skin softer than ordinary soap does by avoiding excessive removal of lipids from the skin surface, but they suffer from the same pH problem.

Most hygiene products contain ingredients called **surfactants** (or sometimes **detergents**). The terms include a wide range of substances, all of which are effective to a greater or lesser degree in dispersing greasy materials in water. Scientists call these materials **hydrophobic**, from the Greek words meaning 'water-hating' because greases will not mix with water unless 'helped' by a surfactant. Soaps are surfactants, strictly speaking, but the term is usually kept specifically for man-made (synthetic) surfactants.

Surfactants are found in laundry detergents, liquid cleansers, shampoos and shower products. Their chemistry makes it possible for them to remove soiling from many different materials, including skin and hair, so that grease and grime can be rinsed away. Some surfactants are harsh to the skin while others are very mild, depending on their type. Only the very gentlest surfactants are incorporated in products for use on human skin.

Surfactants are classified according to their structure:

- **cationic surfactants** (ammonium compounds): these are poorly tolerated by most people's skins, and are now hardly used at all in skin care products
- **anionic surfactants** such as sodium lauryl sulphate – their molecules have a negatively charged 'head' and a long hydrophobic 'tail'; these are widely used because of their good lathering and detergent properties
- **amphoteric surfactants** such as the betaines, and alkylamino acids – these are well tolerated and lather well, and are used in shampoos
- **non-ionic surfactants** such as sucrose esters – overall these molecules are uncharged; these are tolerated better than other types, but do not lather particularly well.

Syndets (short for 'synthetic detergents') are mixtures of synthetic surfactants, mainly anionic surfactants with some added amphoteric surfactants to improve their tolerability. Their potential lies in the fact that their pH may be adjusted to that of skin, and they can be enriched with oily compounds.

To best maintain the skin surface's physiological balance, it may be advisable to use syndets rather than soaps for all personal cleansing. This is especially true for young children, whose skin is more delicate than adult skin. It is also true for the sensitive skin of the scalp, for which the best care centres on the use of a mild shampoo formulated for frequent use.

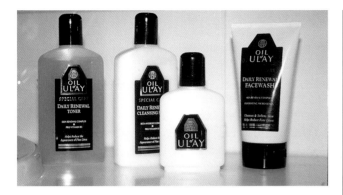

Cleansers and other skin care products come in many forms to meet different needs.

All modern well-formulated cleansing products are based on synthetic detergents.

HOW OFTEN SHOULD WE CLEAN OUR SKIN?

Some people clean their skin only rarely: others are almost obsessive, and go through an elaborate ritual several times a day. (In just the same way, people vary widely in the frequency with which they wash their hair – anything from once a week to twice daily.)

Regular cleaning should not damage the skin *provided* that the products used are well formulated and mild to the skin, and that any extra needs such as dryness are catered for with the regular use of moisturisers.

These needs of course change with time, as the effects of intrinsic and extrinsic ageing become apparent.

Choosing a cleanser

Cleansing should be effective without irritating the skin, and to achieve this it is important to choose the most appropriate products. The following points must be considered when choosing:

- skin type
- age
- any skin problems present
- skin allergies.

Several forms of cleanser have been developed to deal with cleansing different skin types, and to avoid drying the skin as traditional bar soaps tended to do.

Cream, milk or lotion cleansers are particularly suitable for removing make-up and other solid residues from dry skin. All these are **emulsions** (see page 102): they use the dissolving action of oils to remove make-up and other products left on the skin's surface. At the same time they can be formulated to leave behind a moisturising (emollient) film, which prevents too drastic a removal of fats from the skin.

Cleansers should remove oils and other fatty secretions from the sebaceous glands in the skin, but at the same time they should not remove from the stratum corneum the natural lipids like **ceramides**, which have an important role in preventing an excessive loss of water from the skin.

Cleansers for dry skin

In cleansing dry skin the most important aspect is total removal of products. Cleansing products may be spread on the skin surface with the fingers or a pad, and then wiped from the skin with a tissue or rinsed off with water. Manufacturer's instructions must be followed carefully.

Products use the solvent effect of ingredients such as mineral oils and syndets to dissolve make-up and dirt present on the skin, and contain moisturising ingredients as well.

Cleansers for oily skin

Oily (greasy) skin is particularly common in young people, and may be accompanied by an acne condition. One small advantage of having greasy skin is that it tends to be less easily damaged than dry skin, and less prone to moisture loss. It requires less protection in cold weather; a light oil-in-water emulsion is all that is needed.

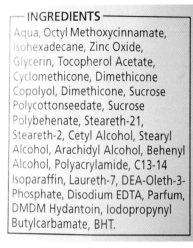

- INGREDIENTS -
Aqua, Octyl Methoxycinnamate, Isohexadecane, Zinc Oxide, Glycerin, Tocopherol Acetate, Cyclomethicone, Dimethicone Copolyol, Dimethicone, Sucrose Polycottonseedate, Sucrose Polybehenate, Steareth-21, Steareth-2, Cetyl Alcohol, Stearyl Alcohol, Arachidyl Alcohol, Behenyl Alcohol, Polyacrylamide, C13-14 Isoparaffin, Laureth-7, DEA-Oleth-3-Phosphate, Disodium EDTA, Parfum, DMDM Hydantoin, Iodopropynyl Butylcarbamate, BHT.

Surfactants form part of many cosmetic products: this one contains sucrose esters (non-ionic surfactants).

Surfactants and the skin

When a cleanser, or any other surfactant product, is rinsed from the skin, slight deposits of surfactant tend to remain. Even some of the less aggressive surfactants can cause a temporary disruption of the keratin protein, eventually leading to increased water loss from the stratum corneum. Repeated surfactant exposure leads to increased water loss. Some surfactants can also damage the lipid structures or even strip them out. This also interferes with the barrier function of the skin so that significant amounts of water may be lost, and the skin can become dry and even flaky.

People with sensitive, type I skins are particularly vulnerable to irritation by harsh surfactants, particularly around the delicate skin of the eyes (see page 146).

The essential requirement of cleansing oily skin is to remove excess surface sebum without total removal of the skin lipids. Severe degreasing treatment can lead to an apparent worsening of sebum secretion, which defeats the aim of the cleansing.

A method of cleansing this type of skin is to wash with a solution of a very mild synthetic detergent (surfactant, see below) containing no oils, waxes or any other lipid agent that could aggravate the oily condition of the skin, sometimes combined with a toning lotion. This kind of product eliminates the oily residue and debris from the skin surface. Some cleansing products contain low concentrations of hydroxy acids (see page 81), which remove dead cells from the upper levels of the stratum corneum. They must be used on a regular basis to work adequately. A light moisturiser may be included in the product to counteract any drying effects of the cleanser.

Facial scrubs

A facial scrub is a light cream containing very fine particles that cleanse the skin by mild abrasion, removing dead cells and dirt. The scrub may be used on greasy skin but should be used with great caution on dry or sensitive skin: where there is doubt, professional skin care advice should be sought. The product is mixed with a small amount of water, applied and massaged in with the fingertips and rinsed off with water.

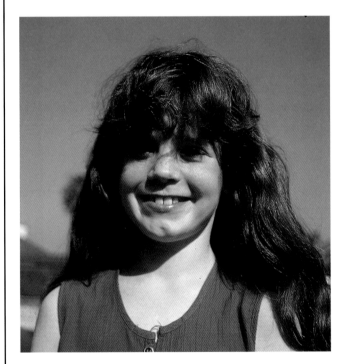

People like this, who have sensitive type I skins, may be particularly vulnerable to skin irritations to surfactants.

Personal cleansing products are now formulated by leading cosmetic manufacturers to be mild but still effective. They are provided in forms that can be used at the basin or in the

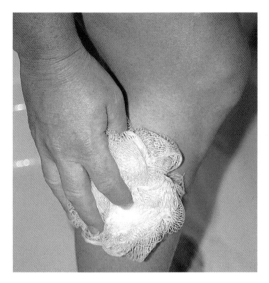

Modern skin care products combine gentle cleansing agents (syndets) with moisturising ingredients. Application in the shower using a 'puff' has a mildly exfoliating action and forms an increasing part of body care for many people.

shower, and often incorporate moisturising ingredients that are deposited on the skin whilst showering.

Measuring the mildness of cleansers

A recognised method of assessing whether a product will irritate the skin is the **Forearm Controlled Application Test** (FCAT).

This involves using an exaggerated washing procedure to measure irritation for five consecutive days. The dryness and/or redness of the skin is recorded on day 1, using a standardised scale, and again on day 5. Measurements of skin hydration are taken at the same time.

The results can be compared with the results for a known mild surfactant product.

Toners

Skin toners are used after cleansing to ensure complete removal from the skin of all cleansing preparations, and also after a face mask to remove all traces of the mask. They are based on plant extracts; those for people with oily skin can contain up to 20% of alcohol. **Astringents** are strongly acting toners with a high alcohol content, which may irritate sensitive skins.

INCI name	Function
Aqua (water)	Solvent
Sodium laureth sulfate	Mild cleansing and lathering
Glycine soja	Moisturiser/occlusive
Sodium lauroamphoacetate	Mild cleansing and lathering
PEG-6 caprylic/capric glycerides	Moisturiser/emollient
Palm kernel acid	Thickener/skin conditioner
Magnesium sulfate	Thickener
Glycerin	Moisturiser/humectant
Cocamide MEA	Mild cleansing and lathering
Citric acid	Adjusts pH
Maleated soybean oil	Moisturiser/emollient/occlusive
Parfum	Fragrance
Polyquaternium-10	Skin conditioner and emollient
Disodium EDTA	Chelator
Sodium benzoate	Preservative
DMDM hydantoin	Preservative
BHT	Preservative

Typical formulation of a cleanser with moisturising ingredients. The use by consumers of this kind of product in the shower is increasing.

Moisturisers

As we have seen, even normal skin needs protection from the effects of simply living. Ageing, the sun, the general environment, all take their toll.

Acquiring the habit of moisturising the skin, particularly with a product that contains a sun protection ingredient, is perhaps the most useful thing to be learnt in cosmetic care.

If the skin is to remain smooth and supple, it needs to maintain an adequate moisture level. It is constantly losing its natural moisture, however, through the epidermis by TEWL. This water loss is aggravated by:

- exposure to the elements – sun, wind, cold
- excessive use of degreasing products on the skin
- central heating and air conditioning
- sebum flow slowing down with age.

What is a moisturiser?

A moisturiser is a product that hydrates the skin, and/or protects the skin from dehydration. That is, it is designed to improve water retention in the epidermis, particularly in the stratum corneum.

Moisturisers are primarily intended to help the skin to function properly in conditions of cold and wind. They are usually creams, of a consistency that varies from light to heavy depending on their content of oil and glycerol. These creams are essentially **oil-in-water emulsions**, consisting of tiny droplets of oil held in a watery base, rather like salad dressings: in these emulsions the watery part is called the **continuous phase**. Salad dressings, however, separate rapidly into their watery and oily constituents; moisturisers, on the other hand, must not separate out even during long-term storage. So part of the skill for a specialist in the formulation of a top-class moisturiser lies in the ability to create a formula that can hold the oil in the water base for a long time without separation or deterioration. This is done by the

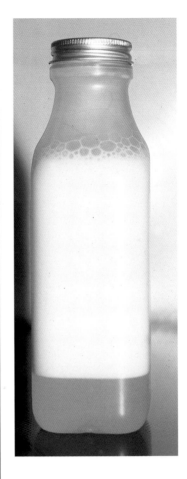

This bottle originally contained an oil-in-water (o/w) emulsion, but the important oily ingredients have separated out from the watery part. Part of the skill of the cosmetic manufacturer lies in producing a stable product that can last for many months.

incorporation of approved and safe **stabilising ingredients**.

An alternative type of moisturiser is a **water-in-oil emulsion**, in which the oily part forms the continuous phase. These are heavier and more greasy, and are aesthetically more suitable for use on the dry skin of the hands, as more of the product remains on the skin and minimises the loss of barrier lipids on subsequent washing or sweating. Skilful formulators can produce water-in-oil (w/o) emulsions with a high proportion of water. Most people find them pleasanter to use than greasier products.

Modern oil-in-water emulsions can be considered for use on dry skin, particularly on the face, where the greasy nature of water-in-oil products may be found unpleasant. Oil-in-water emulsions penetrate well into the skin and can have a cooling effect. Their hydrating effect can be improved by the inclusion in the mixture of 1–2% of urea, which is naturally found in skin.

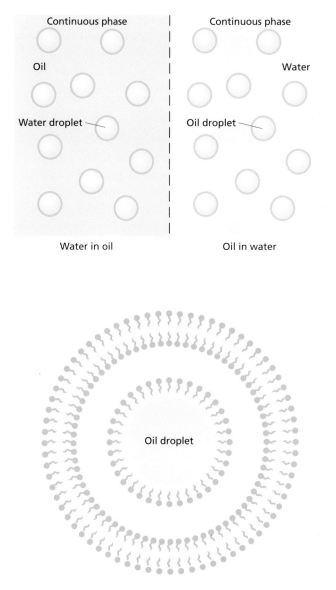

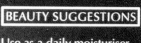

Emulsions: (above) the two types of emulsion; (below) an oil droplet in water, surrounded by a ring of stabiliser molecules that prevent it from coalescing with its neighbours.

Most moisturisers contain substances called **humectants**. These are substances that are capable of attracting water, and which so help to conserve the water in the skin. One of the oldest and best examples is glycerine, also called glycerol. This has been the standard humectant for many decades and is regarded as completely safe.

Because most cosmetic moisturising products have a water base they must contain

preservatives, in order to protect them from being contaminated by bacteria, moulds and yeasts. These micro-organisms are everywhere, in the environment as well as on and in our bodies. Without preservatives, micro-organisms would rapidly spoil the product, and even cause it to become a health hazard. Well-formulated products are likely to contain preservatives, although only tiny amounts are required. The preservatives used are all well known and their concentrations carefully controlled. Parabens are common examples.

Moisturisers for daily use

We have only to look at the cosmetics counters in the shops to see how many different types of moisturiser are available. Skilled chemists formulate these products with care to find the best combinations for different types of skin and to meet specific needs.

Nearly all cosmetics contain small amounts of essential preservatives: in this moisturiser two of the parabens are used.

BEAUTY SUGGESTIONS

Use as a daily moisturiser, gently and uniformly massaging into face and neck area. For personalised skincare advice, call our beauty consultant on FREEPHONE 0800 708708.

Caution: Avoid eye contact. If product gets into the eyes rinse thoroughly with water.

INGREDIENTS
Aqua, Octyl Methoxycinnamate, Isohexadecane, Butylene Glycol, Glycerin, Cetyl Alcohol, TEA Phenylbenzimidazole Sulphonate, Cetyl Phosphate, TEA Palmitate, Aluminium Starch Octenylsuccinate, Titanium Dioxide, TEA Carbomer, Cetyl Palmitate, TEA Stearate, Acrylates\C10-30 Alkyl Acrylates Cross Polymer, PEG-10 Soya Sterol, Parfum, Disodium EDTA, Ricinus Communis, Imidazolidinyl Urea, Methylparaben, Propylparaben, BHT, C.I 14700, C.I 19140.

For instance, a heavy-duty moisturiser for the hands will contain a large proportion of a humectant such as glycerol. Under normal conditions, however, this would be too heavy for use on the face, and a lighter formulation would be more appropriate.

A cosmetic moisturiser designed to encourage skin hydration will be made up from a small percentage of water and humectant, blended with oils and emulsified to form a liquid or cream. **Night creams** can be water-in-oil emulsions as they contain a high proportion of excellent humectants.

The general rule is that the drier the skin and its environment, the richer should be the moisturiser.

Younger people tend to prefer lighter moisturising products than older generations. This is because the younger the skin, the greater is its capacity to retain water, and the more sebum it produces.

Specialised moisturisers

Cosmetic companies are now producing skin care products that incorporate substances giving protection against ultraviolet radiation, as well as other ingredients for hydration and exfoliation. Products with sunscreens are intended for regular daily use, not only for application during heat waves or on beach holidays.

As we saw in Chapter 4, there is a good deal of scientific evidence that the daily use of a moisturiser with sunscreen ingredients can reduce the long-term effects of photodamage.

Increasingly men, as well as women, are recognising the need for regular moisturising and the daily use of sunscreens.

How a moisturiser may change the appearance of the skin

As we saw earlier (page 28), the way in which visible light interacts with skin is fundamental to how we see it and judge its condition.

There are several ways in which cosmetic preparations may improve the appearance of the skin. Application of a simple oil-in-water emulsion containing glycerol will smooth down the squames and produce swelling of the stratum corneum. This mechanism is responsible for the surface-smoothing effect that

INCI name	Function	INCI name	Function
Aqua (water)	Solvent	Cetyl alcohol	Thickener/stabiliser
Octyl methoxycinnamate	Sunscreen (chemical)	Stearyl alcohol	Emulsifier
Glycerin	Skin conditioning agent/ humectant	Arachidyl alcohol	Emulsifier
		Behenyl alcohol	Emulsifier
Zinc oxide	Sunscreen (physical)	Polyacrylamide	Stabiliser
Isohexadecane	Emollient	C13-14 isoparaffin	Emollient
Isopropyl palmitate	Emollient	Laureth-7	Emulsifier
Tocopherol acetate	Vitamin E	DEA-oleth-3-phosphate	Emollient
Dimethicone	Skin feel agent	Disodium EDTA	Chelator
Dimethiconol	Skin feel agent	Parfum	Fragrance
Sucrose polycottonseedate	Emollient	DMDM hydantoin	Preservative
Sucrose polybehenate	Emollient	Iodopropynyl butylcarbamate	Preservative
Steareth-21	Thickener/stabiliser		
Steareth-2	Thickener/stabiliser	BHT	Stabiliser

The ingredients of a modern, good-quality moisturiser and their functions.

can be seen and felt within minutes after application of a moisturiser to the skin.

In dry stratum corneum only 13–30% of light is transmitted back directly – i.e. at least 60% is scattered. With increasing hydration the stratum corneum becomes more translucent, until transmission of light can reach almost 100%. The amount of visible light directly reaching and returning from melanin and the dermis through the epidermis is much increased. This is responsible for the apparent enhancement of skin colour that is often visible immediately after applying a moisturiser.

Untreated skin always carries a certain amount of surface debris ('rubbish') called **detritus** such as loose skin cells (squames). Glycerol and the oils in moisturisers tend to 'paste down' these irregularities on the skin surface, so increasing its reflectance and reducing the appearance of surface roughness.

Continued application of a moisturising product will decrease stratum corneum turnover time, due to the improved efficiency of the desquamation process. This will result in less surface debris and hence better reflectance, together with a thinner, more compact stratum corneum.

Hand creams

Hand creams are used for the purposes of cosmetic skin care, for skin protection and for medical care in people who suffer from hand eczema or irritant dermatitis.

Eczema of the hands is one of the most common skin disorders. It is a particularly troublesome occupational disease; before the introduction of washing machines into most homes it used to be known as housewife's eczema. Eczema of the hands can increase the risk of allergic dermatitis since the damaged skin loses its barrier function, and substances that can cause allergies (**allergens**), such as nickel, can more easily penetrate the skin and sensitize it. Many sufferers from the condition experience repeated outbreaks of hand eczema because the skin of their hands is frequently penetrated by alkaline and irritating solutions over many years. After many such attacks sensitization to particular chemicals and allergic contact dermatitis may develop, frequently only after several years. In some people the condition becomes so severe that they become unable to work.

Irritant substances are of many kinds, including soaps and other harsh surfactants. These substances play a significant role in hand eczema. Washing, even with nothing but water, reduces the water-binding capacity of the stratum corneum, and washing with surfactant solutions has an even more marked effect. Surfactants penetrate the stratum corneum, disrupting the lipid 'brick' structure, and tend to remove the lipid film on the skin surface. As a result, the substances capable of binding water

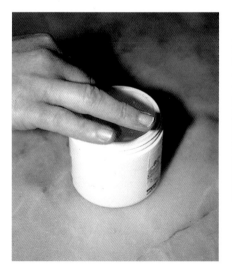 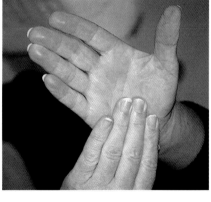 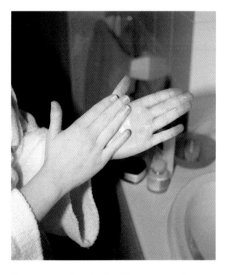

Hand care is vital to protect the epidermis from repeated washing, trauma and occupational abuse. Water-in-oil creams are gradually being supplemented by high-quality oil-in-water products.

Even those hands that have never been traumatised by wet work need care to maintain their attractiveness.

are then easily washed out of the stratum corneum. This is why washing has such a dehydrating effect. As well as removing the skin surface lipids, surfactants can also remove the lipids of sebum (although these are not particularly important in the skin of the hands). One of the most important reasons for using a hand cream is to protect the skin by reducing the penetration of irritants.

Cosmetic hand creams that are of value are o/w emulsions with a high water content, often more than 60%. Nearly all cosmetic hand creams contain substances that bind water, particularly glycerol, sorbitol and propylene glycol, as well as preservatives. Other important components are skin protection substances, especially silicone oils and substances based on them, and hydrophobic fatty acid esters. These are thought to form a protective film on the skin after the lipid component has been penetrated and the water evaporated. Vaseline, liquid paraffin and other hydrophobic lipids would be expected to have a similar effect.

Specialised **skin protection products** can be either water-in-oil or oil-in-water emulsions. Water-in-oil emulsions can be used to provide protection against hydrophilic ('water-loving') irritants, which include soaps and detergents, and also acids and bases, oil coolants, and so on. They also show a good skin care effect. Their use does not involve significant risk of lipid removal from the skin, because the emulsifiers they contain cannot emulsify lipids in water. Unfortunately the skin can feel sticky after their use, and they are not particularly popular among consumers.

Even such specialised products cannot completely protect the skin against all irritants, however.

Body lotions and bath oils

Body lotions and bath oils are used by doctors to help eczema patients, but are increasingly popular even among people whose skin is not dry because they soften and smooth the skin.

Dry and rough skin is found in atopic people, those with eczema and the elderly. It is probable that in most of these people the condition of

the skin is accentuated by washing with unnecessarily harsh products, because soaps and detergents remove sebaceous gland lipids from the skin. The most important feature of daily skin care is a reduction of this wash damage. Body lotions and bath oils can offer further help.

Body lotions are emulsions that have been formulated so as to minimise any drying effect. Water-in-oil emulsions are particularly useful for use on dry skin, as they remain on the skin and reduce removal of barrier lipids on subsequent washing or sweating. Water-in-oil emulsions with a high proportion of water are useful, since they are well absorbed into the skin and more pleasant to use.

When body lotions are used by people with a normal skin, the requirements for the emulsions are less important.

Bath oils are of two types:

- spreading bath oils
- emulsion bath oils.

Spreading bath oils do not contain surfactants. They produce lipid films that float on the surface of the bath water, and spread on to the surface of the skin when the user leaves the bath. The cooler the bath water, the better is the lipid coverage of the skin. Overall, a spreading bath oil has as beneficial an effect as a w/o-type body lotion.

Emulsion bath oils, on the other hand, do contain surfactants. They emulsify the lipids in the bath water, and have a relatively good

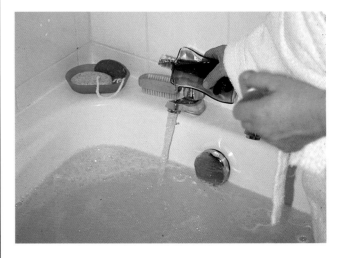

A spreading oil – useful for dry skin, especially for children.

cleansing effect. People with dry skin should restrict themselves to using only bath oils that contain small amounts of surfactants. People with normal skin, however, should not experience any negative effects even where the surfactant levels are quite high.

Some special ingredients of skin care products

Antioxidants

The antioxidants used in cosmetics are derived from certain vitamins, mainly A, C and E, which form part of the body's natural defence and balance system. Antioxidants are thought to protect the skin by attaching themselves to free radicals, minimising the harm they do to the skin. These additives may help the skin repair systems, but hard scientific evidence for this is limited.

D-Panthenol

This substance is readily converted into vitamin B5, which has been shown to help the skin to repair damage.

Vitamin E

This is commonly included in cosmetics. It may help to reduce the effects of free radicals formed from sun damage.

Pro-vitamin A

This is another antioxidant that may help to reduce the effects of free radicals.

Hyaluronic acid

As we have seen (page 30), this natural moisturiser forms part of the tissue that surrounds the collagen and elastin fibres.

As we age, we produce less hyaluronic acid in our skin, which becomes less resilient and pliable. Hyaluronic acid is often added to moisturisers, and can be injected by doctors into the skin.

Ceramides

These are lipids that help to prevent moisture loss through the skin. They assist the skin in its function as an efficient barrier.

Retinoic acid

This is a derivative of vitamin A which was originally prescribed in high doses for the treatment of acne. It does refine the skin, increase collagen production and reduce wrinkles, but it can have unpleasant side-effects such as extreme sensitivity to sunlight, with increased reddening of the skin and peeling. It is available on prescription from a dermatologist for severe sun damage. Well-formulated cosmetics may contain moderate and harmless amounts of retinoic acid derivatives, which at these levels have some hydrating effects.

Liposomes

Liposomes are tiny, hollow spheres of lipids (fats), which are filled with active ingredients. They are designed as a transportation system to carry these ingredients to the places where the skin needs them. Liposome spheres are smaller than skin cells, therefore ingredients held inside them can be delivered with great accuracy into the skin and released precisely as needed.

Nanospheres

These are smaller versions of liposomes. Because of their smaller size, they are supposed to penetrate deeper into the skin.

SKIN MYTH

Many cosmetic creams have an anti-ageing effect because they contain the proteins collagen and/or elastin.

Fact: Collagen forms fibres in the dermis which give the skin structural support, provide strength, and allow the skin to stretch and contract. Elastin is the protein that binds the collagen bundles together. Despite the name, we do not know whether elastin is actually responsible for the skin's elasticity.

When applied to the skin, these creams do not have much effect on the changes in appearance due to natural ageing. They do have humectant properties, however, plumping out the skin with retained moisture.

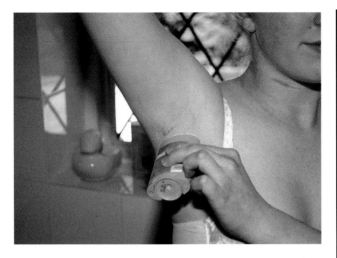

Underarm care. Antiperspirants control sweat activity and the growth of the bacteria that cause body odour.

Deodorants and antiperspirants

Unpleasant body odour has become as socially unacceptable as bad breath. It is not surprising, therefore, that there is a lot of evidence to show that underarm care is important for social confidence.

Use of underarm products to reduce body odour amongst women in north-western Europe and North America approaches 100%: in southern Europe the figure is nearer to 75%. Usage amongst men is close to 85% in the USA and northern Europe but only about 60% in southern Europe. There is no hard evidence to explain these cultural differences.

The most commonly expressed needs in underarm care are for products that effectively protect against odour and wetness, that do not irritate the skin and that have all-day efficacy.

Control of body odour (often shortened to 'BO') necessitates daily usage of antiperspirant or deodorant products from puberty onwards. Bacteria play a significant role in malodour formation. Thorough washing of the armpit can reduce germs by more than 99%; unfortunately, the few that survive washing grow very rapidly and their numbers return to the previous high level in a few hours.

Continued, daily use of an antiperspirant can be highly effective in controlling body odour. Interaction of sweat with the active ingredient of the antiperspirant leads to superficial plugging of those sweat ducts that are currently producing sweat. The plugs formed are gradually lost over several days (between two and four) through the natural skin shedding process.

Modern well-formulated antiperspirants offer a logical and significant benefit to quality of life. Reduction of malodour and wetness enhance individual social confidence.

The antiperspirants available today are very safe products. The incidence of irritation reactions is low, even though they are normally applied to the skin in an area that is quite sensitive, and which may have been shaved. Scientists can now calculate the amount of ingredients likely to be deposited in a lifetime. There is no evidence that using such products over long periods has any side-effects on the body.

DEODORANT OR ANTIPERSPIRANT?

Deodorants contain an antibacterial agent and fragrance: triclocarbon and triclosan are the main antibacterial agents used in deodorant formulations today.

Antiperspirants reduce sweating and dramatically alter the favourable environment in which bacteria grow. Aluminium chlorohydrate and aluminium zirconium glycine complex salts are the most commonly used active ingredients in antiperspirant products marketed today.

Additional products

In this section we look at some additional types of product that are beneficial to the proper working of the skin at various ages.

Personal preference is important in the choice of product. Within the range of available choices, it is the responsibility of the cosmetic industry to provide logical and good-quality products.

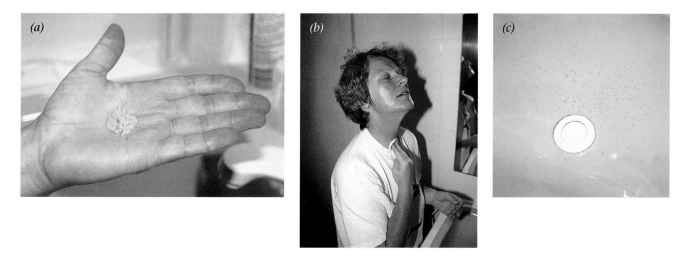

Exfoliation: (a) only a little product is needed; (b) the cream is applied carefully but thoroughly; (c) the removal of dead squames leaves the skin feeling smooth.

Exfoliators

These gently and effectively remove dead cells from the skin's surface by mechanical means, thus removing surface debris They are suitable for greasy or normal skin, but should be used with caution on dry or sensitive skin. If in doubt seek professional skin care advice.

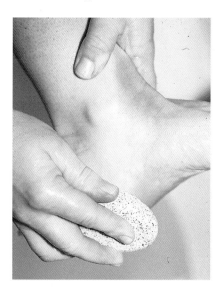

Treating the feet with pumice – a traditional method of removing dead squames from the soles of the feet by gentle abrasion. Here the stratum corneum is at its thickest. This remains a popular method of removing excessive dead skin.

Mud packs

These seem to help with spots and so-called 'deep cleaning'. They are especially suitable for greasy skin, but may be compatible with most skin types.

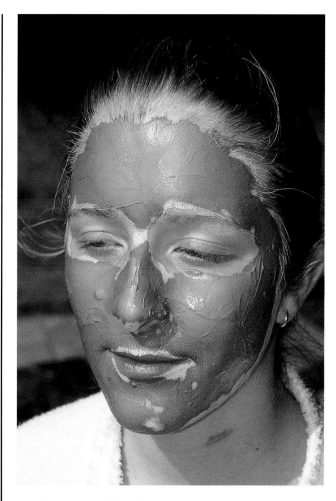

A facial mask works well for really deep cleansing – that is, cleansing that penetrates deep into the sebaceous duct, not into the epidermis.

SUMMARY OF PRODUCTS USED IN A TYPICAL SKIN CARE ROUTINE

- cleansers
- make-up remover
- toner
- day and night moisturisers
- anti-wrinkle creams
- special products such as eye area lotions
- hand creams
- antiperspirants.

Bar soap is acceptable if the skin is very greasy, but the product chosen must be a well-formulated one. The aesthetic effects of using soap also depend on the degree of hardness of the local water.

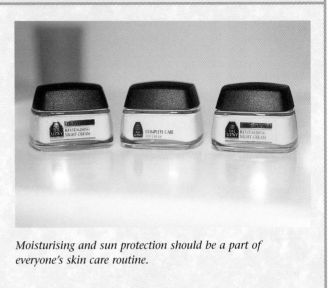

Moisturising and sun protection should be a part of everyone's skin care routine.

Cold compresses

These useful traditional remedies reduce puffiness – see the photograph on page 12 – and are especially useful around the eye area.

Hot compresses

These can be invaluable and safe aids for troublesome spots. Their use is far preferable to squeezing, the trauma of which may lead to scarring.

Differences in societies

The way different peoples look after their skin is often dictated by the degree of affluence.

In rural parts of Africa women still make crude bars of soap using crude potassium hydroxide produced from burnt tree bark. Many use coconut oil as a moisturiser.

In addition many women try to lighten their skin by using skin creams containing certain drugs. Steroid creams are freely available for sale in some places, as are creams containing skin-lightening ingredients called **hydroquinones**. In the developed world these ingredients can legally be incorporated in low concentrations in well-formulated cosmetic preparations, but their unrestricted use in poorly formulated products can sometimes produce hideous results.

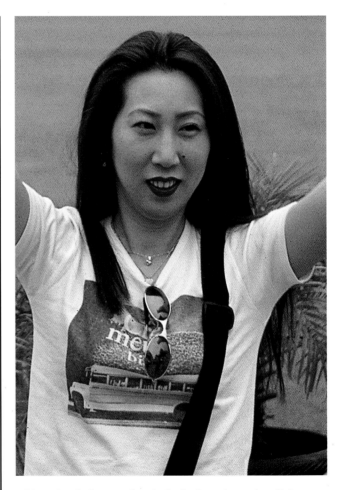

This Asian lady uses chemicals (hydroquinones) to lighten her facial colour. Light skin is regarded as a mark of class, status and wealth in many cultures.

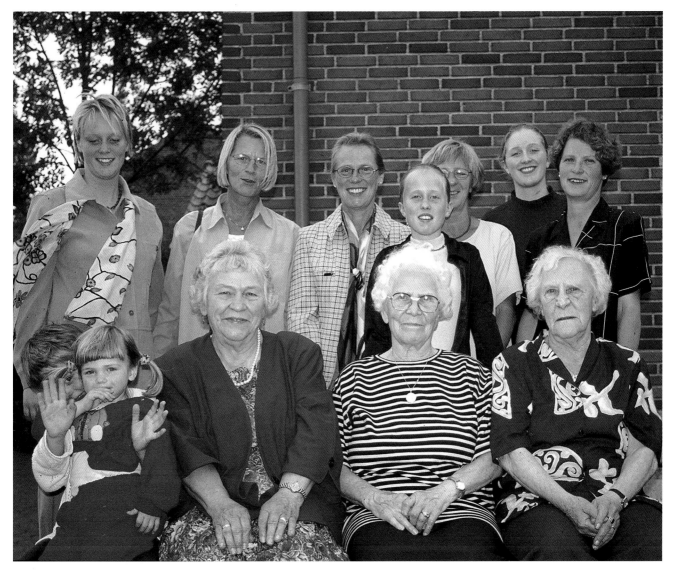

Four generations of one family: from childhood to old age, appropriate skin care is important to them all.

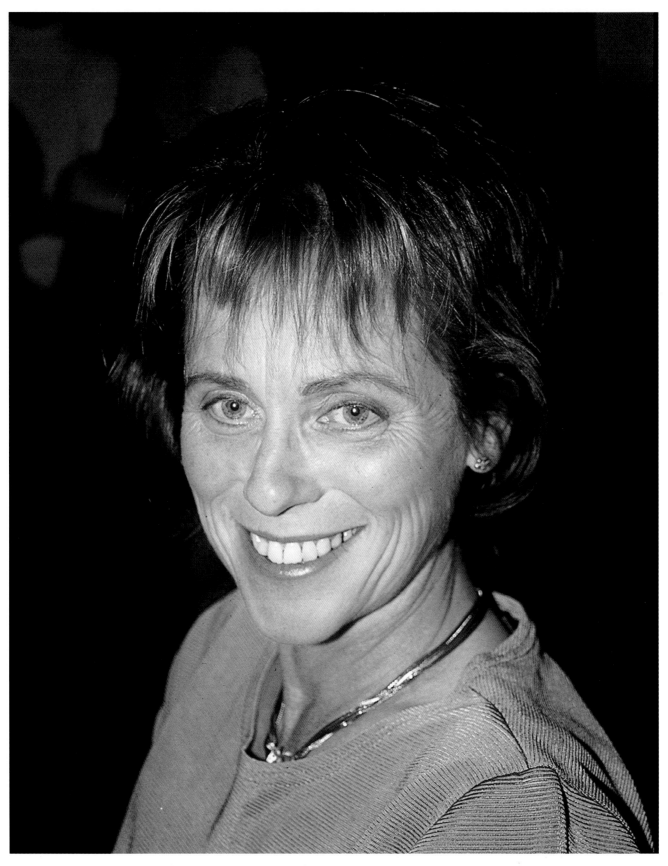

Decorative cosmetics, chosen for a special occasion, enhance what Nature gave.

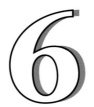

6
Decorative cosmetics

Ever since ancient times, people have used preparations that they hope will change or modify their appearance, particularly that of the face. Ancient Egyptian cosmetics, at least three thousand years old, have been shown to consist of artificially synthesised mineral powders mixed with lipids. Cleopatra, a mere two thousand years ago, is known to have used perfumed ointments, eye make-up and lip colours.

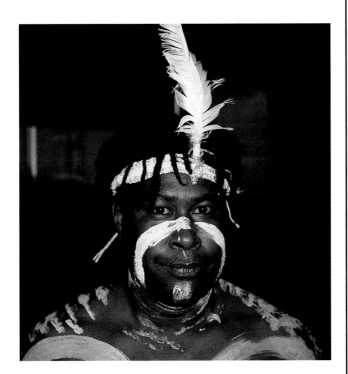

Decorative cosmetics have been used for thousands of years to enhance the appearance. This gentleman's ancestors migrated from south-east Asia to Australasia some forty thousand years ago. He still uses the traditional cosmetics made from mud, which became the forerunners of today's sophisticated products.

So-called decorative cosmetics are intended to enhance certain features, particularly the eyes and the lips, and to conceal undesirable features such as blemishes on the skin of the face and in some countries that of the upper body as well.

There are other factors: in certain cultures white skin is still thought desirable as it is seen as signifying a non-manual way of life and therefore high social standing. Even today some people with dark skins confess they would prefer a lighter hue, as they regard a very dark colour as indicating low-status field work. People with strong opinions of this kind are likely to seek out any cosmetics that claim to lighten or hide their own skin colour.

The use of decorative cosmetics is still concerned with perceived social status, fashion and style copying. The demand for these products has extended the production of decorative cosmetics into a multi-billion pound global business operating primarily, though not exclusively, for women.

The term **cosmetic** means an article intended to be applied to the human body – whether rubbed, poured, sprinkled or sprayed on to it – or to any part of it, for the purposes of cleansing, beautifying, promoting attractiveness or in other ways altering the appearance of the skin.

Today's cosmetic products, however, do more than simply please the user by improving the appearance of the skin. In addition, they can help to improve the physiology and condition of the skin through the activity of certain specialised, safe ingredients that have been developed by the industry's scientists. These effects of cosmetics are only temporary, however; the active ingredients are not drugs. Drugs may influence the activity of the skin's

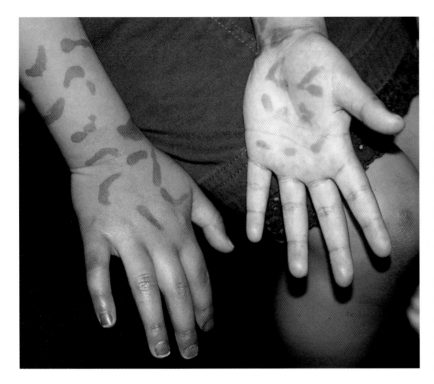

components. The skill of the cosmetic manufacturer lies in the mixing of these ingredients in just the right proportions to remain stable even if stored for a long time and to give pleasure and satisfaction to the user each time the product is applied to the skin. All the modern technology used by the cosmetics industry, all the new ingredients that are developed and the new instrumentation that is used in product evaluation, take second place to this skill.

In this chapter, we shall look at the functions of a range of decorative cosmetics, what they are made of, and how their manufacturers ensure that they are safe, stable, well preserved, and efficacious.

Henna tattoos like these are common hand decorations in some cultures.

cells permanently: for example, a drug might provide a lasting cure for a skin problem. By contrast, although a skin problem might improve after treatment with a cosmetic product it is likely to reappear when treatment stops.

The high-quality products many people seek are the results of the successful combination of a large variety of oils, waxes, humectants, moisturisers, solubilisers, emulsifiers, preservatives, antioxidants and other

Foundations

Foundations are used primarily to improve the appearance of skin texture and to act as a base for other decorative cosmetics. Many foundations still contain talc, for a smooth texture, and other powdery materials chosen for their good covering power: these are useful for hiding tiny blemishes such as freckles. All foundations include some colouring material, to enhance the natural colour of the skin.

Different types of foundation: (left) a powder foundation, (right) a foundation cream.

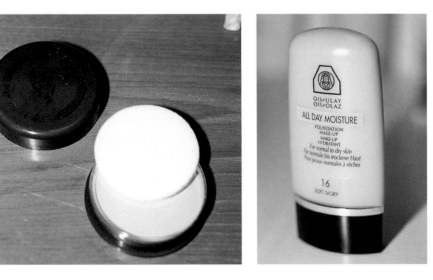

There are many different types of foundation, formulated as cakes, sticks, creams and liquids. Some include moisturisers, and especially benefit dry skin in winter. Others contain useful amounts of sunscreen ingredients.

Cake foundations contain a small amount of surfactant, and when used with a wet sponge they form creamy emulsions that spread smoothly on the face.

Oil-based foundations are marketed in both compact and stick form. The sticks have especially good covering power, useful for camouflaging birthmarks or other skin markings that cannot be hidden by other foundations. These foundations are emollient, and so are especially suitable for use in autumn and winter.

Both oil-in-water and water-in-oil emulsion foundations are available. In the o/w emulsions, the oily ingredients and the solid powders are distributed evenly through the water base, together with a stabiliser for the emulsion. They are formulated as both creams and liquids: the difference lies in the proportion of oil in the mixture and also the amount of powder. Their disadvantage is that they are affected by both sweat and sebum, so that the make-up needs retouching from time to time.

Make-up based on a modern w/o emulsion foundation needs less retouching that the older products and keeps its appearance well through the day.

Some w/o emulsion foundations are unstable, and form two layers on standing and must be well shaken before application. Most people find them pleasant to use for a light make-up in summer. A solid form of w/o emulsion is available, which is basically a cream foundation to which has been added a proportion of wax.

The choice of foundation is a highly individual one, and in the end is a matter of personal preference. Both the skin type and the season of the year need to be borne in mind before a final decision is made. It is often worth buying tiny sample containers with which to experiment first.

Face powders

Face powders have been in use for centuries for the purpose of changing the colour of the face to make it more attractive, and particularly to cover up minor blemishes. Nowadays foundation make-up fulfils these functions, and the main use of powders today is to remove the oily shine due to sweat and sebum and keep the makeup looking good for longer. They can also subtly change the skin colour, and give an effect similar to that of rouge.

Face powders are made in various forms. In **loose powder**, almost all the raw materials is talc to enable smooth application. Coloured and pearly pigments are added to enhance the skin colour. Loose powder is usually applied with a puff on top of emulsion or oil-based foundations to achieve a matt, clear skin colour.

Pressed (compact) powder has similar functions to those of loose powder. Many people prefer to use loose powder in the home, keeping compact powder for touching up make-up when away from home. The materials used to make compact powder are basically the same as those for loose powder, together with a little oil as a binding agent.

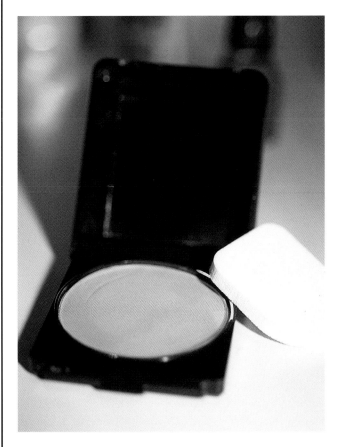

Pressed face powder.

Rouges

Rouges, often known as **blushers**, are products designed to tint the face and mimic a 'healthy' complexion. They are available in the form of powders (loose and compact), sticks, creams and liquids.

Originally all rouges were produced in shades of red or pink, but now the range includes brownish and bluish shades. The base formulae for powder and cream rouges are similar, with talc as the main ingredient of both. Oil-based rouges are essentially a mixture of kaolin, petrolatum, liquid paraffin and pigment.

Eye make-up

Since eye make-up is applied to skin that is perhaps more delicate than that of any other part of the body, as well as lying close to the eyes themselves, it is especially important that it should not cause any skin irritation. The colourings and preservatives used are therefore in highly purified forms. Well-formulated products should also be easy to apply and reasonably permanent. Colouring agents are the major constituents of most cosmetic eye preparations.

Eye make-up products are of three main types:

- those used to enhance the appearance of the eyelashes – **mascaras**
- those used to colour the eyelids and the skin around the eyes – **eye-shadows**, **eyeliners** and **eyebrow make-up**
- those used to reduce the dryness of the thin skin of the eye area, or to remove eye make-up – **eye creams** and **eye make-up removers**.

Most of the colouring materials used are inorganic pigments. Sometimes finely powdered metal, such as aluminium powder, is added to give a metallic or 'glitter' appearance.

Mascaras

Mascaras are pigmented preparations for application to the eyelashes, to make them look darker and longer and to make the whites of the eyes look brighter by contrast. Old-style mascara was applied from a cake, using a wetted brush, but this practice was not entirely hygienic and has almost disappeared. Modern mascaras are creams. Some contain nylon fibres, to produce an apparent lengthening of the lashes.

The basic ingredients are

- oils, mainly the very stable petrolatum or petrolatum distillate
- silicone oils, which improve water resistance and make the mascara more permanent
- waxes
- pigment (usually black, brown or dark blue).

Eye shadows

Eye shadows are preparations applied to the eyelids in order to enhance the 'background' for the eyes and to make the eyes look larger. They may take the form of creams, sticks or powders. The product is applied to the eyelids with a soft dry brush or a foam-tipped applicator.

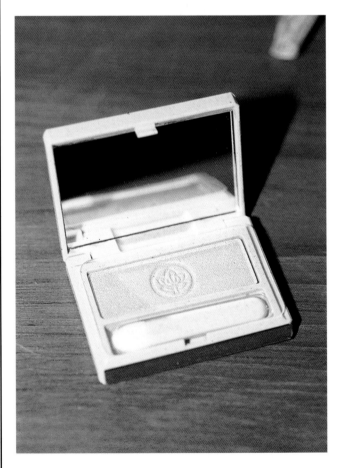

Pressed powder eye shadow.

The basis of a pressed eye shadow is talc (hydrated magnesium silicate), which may form up to half of the product. Talc is used because it has excellent covering power and good slip and smoothness. A special grade of talc is used that is free of asbestos and heavy metals.

Powdered kaolin, titanium dioxide, chalk (calcium carbonate) and potato starch are all used for their covering power. Metallic soaps are essential ingredients, needed to make the shadow adhere to the eyelids. Carefully chosen pigments and preservatives are included in the product as well.

Eyeliners

Eyeliners are cosmetics designed to accentuate the expressiveness of the eyes. They are available in liquid and pencil form, and are generally chosen to harmonise with the shade of the mascara that is being worn. The product will be water-resistant, for permanence in wear.

The basic component is a polymeric material that is a water-thickening agent: those most commonly used include a magnesium aluminium silicate (veegum), poly(vinyl-pyrrolidone) (PVP), acrylic derivatives and cellulose derivatives.

Pigments and preservatives are also included.

Eyebrow make-up

Eyebrow make-up is used in order to change the structure and shape of the eyebrows. An eyebrow pencil can be used to draw in absent eyebrows.

Eyebrow pencils are formed by mixing pigments (generally iron oxides) with waxes (synthetic or natural) and oils to make a composition that glides smoothly on to the skin without dragging it.

Eye creams

These are generally water-in-oil emulsions. They have two functions:

- to reduce dryness of the skin of the eye area by lubricating it
- to provide an adherent base over which eye-shadow can be applied.

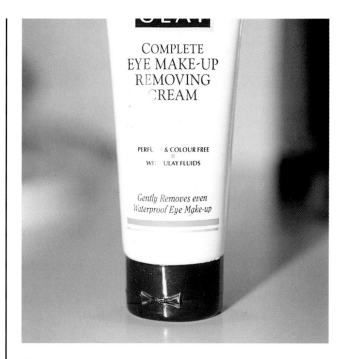

Eye make-up remover cream, formulated so that it can be smoothed on and removed without dragging of the delicate skin of the eye region. It is important that these products are formulated to be gentle so as to prevent irritation to the sensitive skin around the eye. Like all modern cosmetic products, these preparations are tested by dermatologists to ensure safety for consumers (see page 143).

Eye make-up removers

Eye make-up, once applied, must be removed with great care and gentleness. A variety of eye make-up removers has been formulated. The most popular forms are creams and lotions, and remover pads soaked in a lotion.

The basic components of eye make-up removers are oils and mild detergents. The composition of the mixture is carefully designed to be compatible with the delicate skin of the eyelids and the area around the eye.

Lipsticks

In the ancient world Greeks and Romans took plant and animal extracts to apply to the lips and cheeks. Carmine (cochineal), a vivid red pigment extracted from dried bodies of the cochineal beetle found in Mexico, came into use in Europe after the discovery of the Americas.

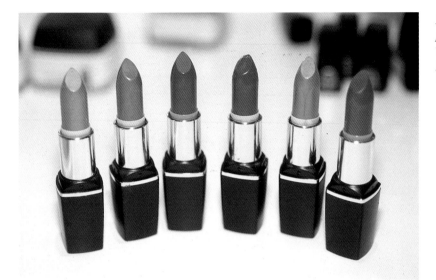

Lipsticks are at the fun end of the cosmetic product range, but they must be formulated with scientific skill and care as well as with fashion knowledge. Modern lipsticks may include moisturising ingredients.

Carthamin, made from sunflowers, was used in Japan.

The lipsticks of today are composed of oils, fats, waxes and pigments. Since about 1940, carmine and carthamin have been replaced with synthetic colours, to which various inorganic pigments are added in order to obtain the wide range of subtle shades that fashion dictates.

Well-formulated lipsticks have a humectant function (see page 103). Some include in their base formula an emulsion that incorporates water and a humectant in stable proportions. Some include UV protectors, and some are even colourless!

Nail varnish

Nail varnish components include lacquer – a complex mixture of resins, solvents, plasticisers and other ingredients – and a suspension base together with pigments, and sometimes pearlescent materials and special additives. These additives may include nylon fibres, acrylics, gelatin and other proteins. All these raw materials are chosen to be non-toxic, non-irritant and non-sensitising to the skin. Whereas choosing and wearing nail varnish should be fun – like child's play – selecting the ingredients for nail varnish is a serious business!

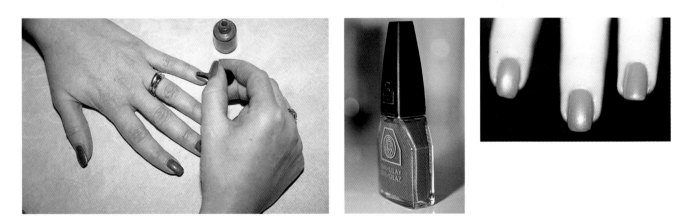

A high-quality nail varnish is easy to apply, and dries and hardens rapidly. It has a vivid colour and shine and a rich gloss, it is waterproof and flexible, adheres well to the nails, and resists chipping and abrasion.

Nail varnish removers

Nail varnish removers are essentially solvents that soften and dissolve old varnish so that it can be wiped away. Most contain acetone or similar compounds. Since they also dissolve lipids, some contain oils to protect the nails from their drying effect.

A few people can experience an allergic reaction or irritant dermatitis to a remover solution. The most modern acetone-based varnish removers are less harsh to the skin because they contain a proportion of water, together with other ingredients to reduce tissue irritation.

Care is needed in handling these solvents, as they can present a fire hazard.

Nail hardeners and strengtheners

Nail hardeners and strengtheners work in two ways: either by penetrating the nail or by providing a strong protective coating.

Formaldehyde is an effective nail hardener, but it is toxic at levels above a certain limit permitted by law. A warning label is required for hardeners containing more than 0.50% free formaldehyde. Formaldehyde probably works by cross-linking some of the nail proteins, resulting in strengthening.

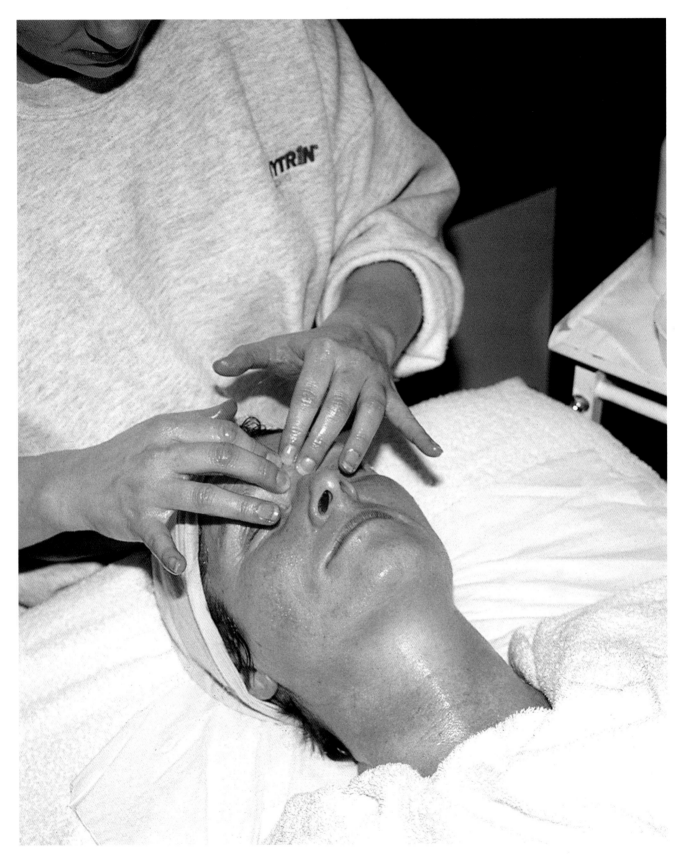

At the beauty salon, the client should be happy to put herself into the hands of an expert beauty therapist. Understanding the science of skin care is important.

7
At the beauty salon

When regular clients come to the salon, it is important to understand the scientific basis for the various treatments they are given. Much of this is discussed elsewhere in this book.

Some processes, however, have little or no scientific basis. One such is the application of total body wraps containing all manner of strange and even absurd ingredients, often exotic and little-known 'herbs', with the intention of removing all the 'toxins' from the body by sweating. These products do indeed produce sweating, help remove sebum from the upper part of the sebaceous glands and may clear skin contaminants.

'Toxins' are another matter, however. Toxins from the scientific standpoint are natural waste products formed in the body from materials we eat, drink or inhale. Almost all of them are dealt with very effectively by the liver and kidneys, which act as the body's natural sewerage plant. The rest are excreted in very tiny amounts via the sebaceous glands. As a result, toxins do not swarm unchecked in the bloodstream and skin: they are not even particularly poisonous.

There is therefore no need to employ special procedures to get rid of toxins. In any case, body masks cannot do so – indeed, if they were indeed able to extract toxins from the blood they would also drag out essential minerals, with disastrous results for health.

At the beauty salon, as in many other circumstances, the use of your scientific knowledge together with some sound common sense will stand you in good stead.

At the beauty therapist's: an illustrated guide

In the rest of this chapter, the types of procedure that are carried out by a qualified beauty therapist are illustrated. The details of an individual routine vary from client to client, and are governed by such factors as skin type and client preference. The therapist's attention and skill can bring some physiological benefits to the hydration and appearance of the skin and for the application of decorative cosmetics, as well as considerable psychological benefit to the client.

The client shown here goes through a series of procedures designed to remove detritus, sebum and dead squames from the skin by cleansing, toning and exfoliation. We have seen how these improve the rate of turnover of skin cells, and how if performed on a regular basis they can reduce the appearance of fine lines.

This is followed by a facial mask treatment, which increases sweating and removes sebum from the upper part of the sebaceous glands, and then by a facial massage. Occlusion with a clay-based mask will improve hydration, and will remove sebum from as deep as possible in the sebaceous duct. We have also seen that massage improves lymph drainage, particularly around the eye area.

After these treatments a foundation is applied as the basis for the application of other decorative cosmetics. Modern foundations make the skin look smoother, cover blemishes and can also help hydration.

Finally a range of decorative cosmetics is applied. These cosmetics enhance the features, particularly those apparently evolved by nature for the attraction of the opposite sex. The eyes and the lips can send out strong signals, and decorative cosmetics change their appearance by enhancing their colour and apparently increasing their size.

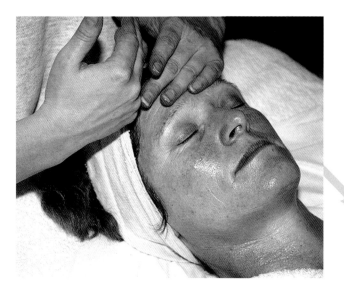

Cleaning removes surface debris including sebum and everyday pollutants. A cleansing milk applied with the fingers is here preferred. The formulation allows penetration into the upper part of the sebaceous glands and removal of sebum from more than just the surface layer.

The cleanser is gently wiped away…

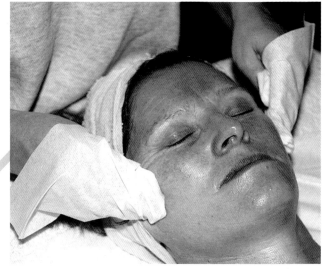

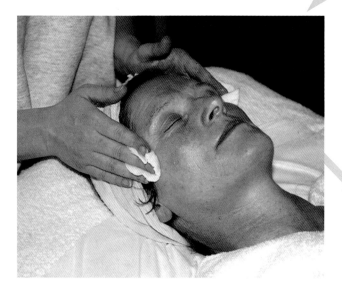

…and a toner applied. Toning removes any residual cleansing material and sebum.

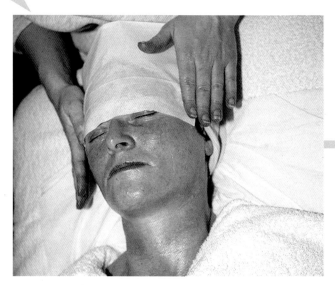

The toner is removed by 'blotting', leaving the face as dry as possible. It leaves the skin feeling clean and fresh by its effect on the nerve endings; it may also temporarily close up the skin pores.

A clay-based mask is spread over the face.

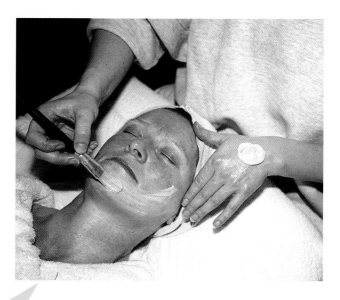

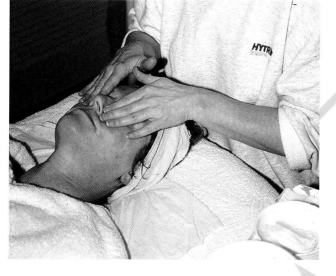

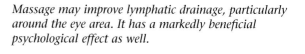

Massage may improve lymphatic drainage, particularly around the eye area. It has a markedly beneficial psychological effect as well.

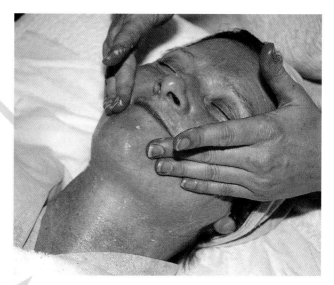

The exfoliant is carefully wiped away, together with the shed dead squames. This is followed by gentle facial massage.

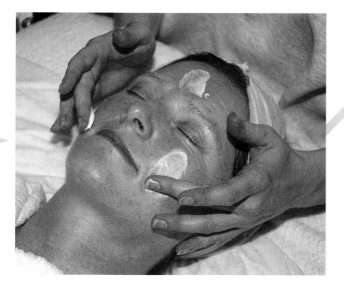

Exfoliation using a fruit acid product removes the surface squames. It improves the surface appearance of the skin and speeds up the regeneration of skin cells. It may contribute to reduction in fine lines.

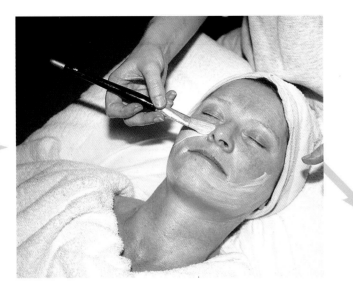

The mask contains ingredients that absorb skin surface lipids. Although their effects are of a temporary nature they improve the appearance of the skin.

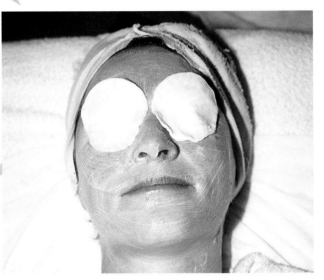

The client relaxes while the mask does its work.

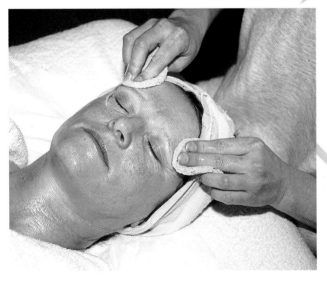

After removing the mask...

...a tinted moisturiser is smoothed into the skin...

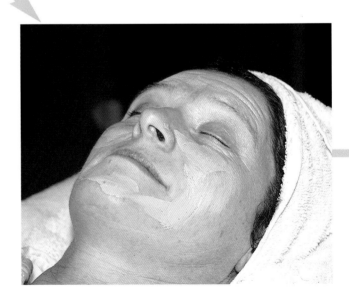

The eyebrows are outlined and emphasised…

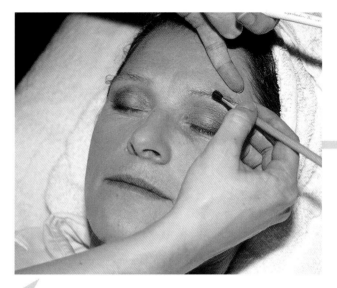

Eye shadow makes the eyes look larger and brighter.

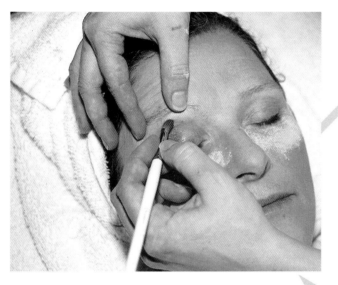

Before decorative cosmetics are applied, the eye area is covered with protective powder.

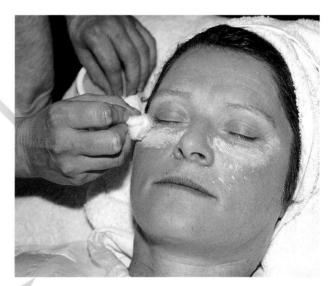

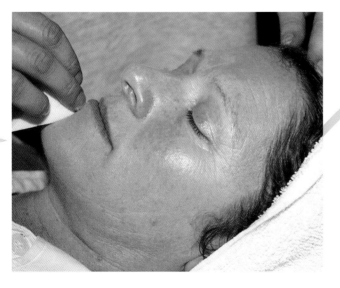

…and a liquid foundation is applied, to provide a basis for the decorative cosmetics. Modern foundations include ingredients that can improve hydration in the stratum corneum.

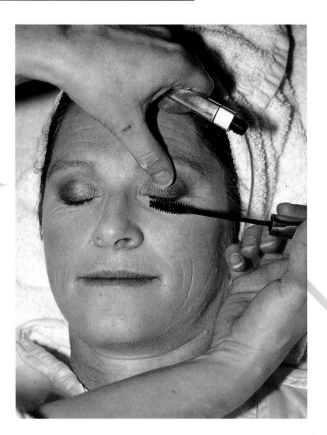

...and the lashes are darkened with mascara to accentuate the eyes.

Lipliner is used to define the outline of the lips...

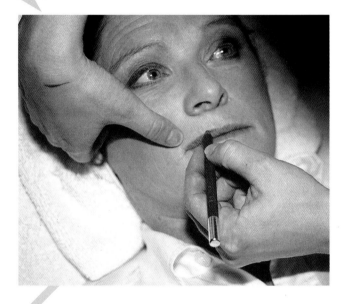

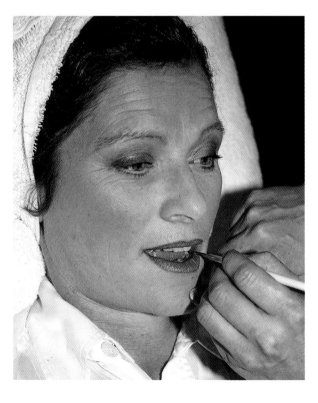

...and a lip brush used to fill the outline with colour.

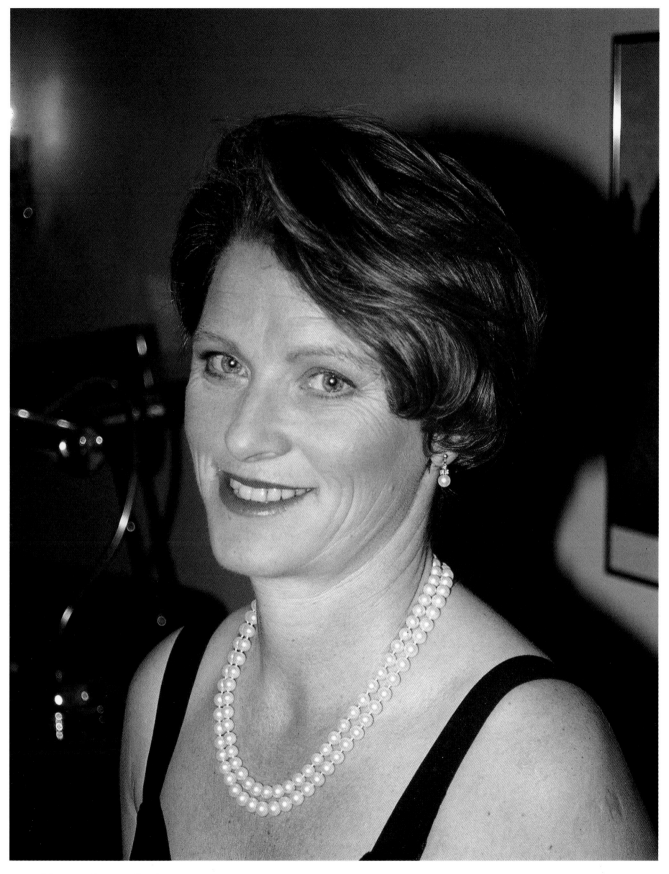

A confident and happy client!

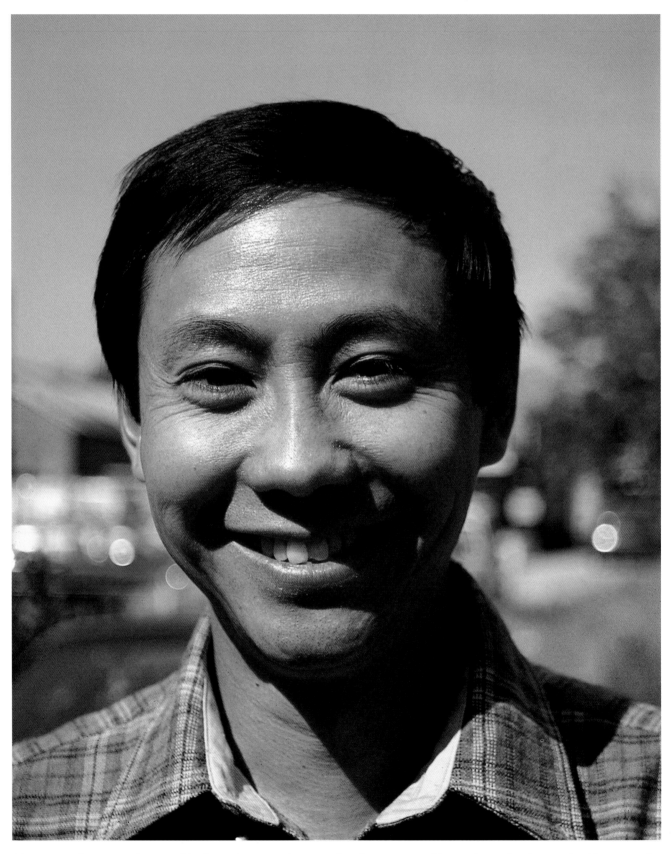

Most men today are not interested in decorative cosmetics, even though many are taking an increasing interest in skin care and protection against the sun.

8

Skin care for men

Cosmetic needs depend on the culture of an individual as a member of a local community, but they are generally far more limited in the male population than in the female.

Cosmetics have traditionally been formulated differently for men and women. Products for men often contain alcohol, which is rarely used in cosmetics for women (except in toners). The appeal to the two groups is also distinct, with men seeking feelings of well-being and health, and women wishing for health and beauty. Men treat their skin in response to a need, such as shaving or cleansing. Not many men currently think of skin care as a way of preventing ageing or a method of improving their appearance.

Men have been conditioned in the past by the availability of a range of products directed towards men only and presented with a masculine orientation.

Their first encounters with these toiletries were generally with shaving products and hair lotions. Aftershaves, antiperspirants and deodorants are increasingly widely used, however, and more men are coming to see the regular use of moisturisers as important. In some countries men are already regularly using sunscreen-containing products.

Cosmetic products made specifically for men include:

- alcoholic perfumery (toilet water and eau de Cologne)
- shaving products
- hair products
- cleansing products.

Shaving and skin care

Masculine needs are largely concentrated on shaving. The beard is a sexual characteristic, which develops with puberty. One of the most important rites marking the transition of a boy into manhood is the first shave.

Most men in our society prefer to be cleanshaven. Since the beard grows 2 mm a day, shaving is a daily necessity.

Shaving repeatedly injures the skin of the face and neck. The razor forcibly removes the surface lipid layer of the skin and the outer layers of the stratum corneum before the cells are ready to be lost by the normal processes of desquamation. This speeds up the turnover of cells, and exposes skin cells that are not yet ready to withstand the effects of the environment.

This harsh treatment of the skin is compounded by the use of high-alcohol-content aftershave lotions, which dissolve even more lipids. Skin cells also become temporarily over-hydrated because of the action of detergents and hot water during shaving. They later lose water, since they have lost so much of the lipids that help them retain moisture. The result can be dry, flaky cells and dull-looking skin. In addition, the skin may begin to feel uncomfortably tight as the outer cells shrink owing to water loss and become, in turn, more sensitive to the irritant effects of sweating, sebum and the environment.

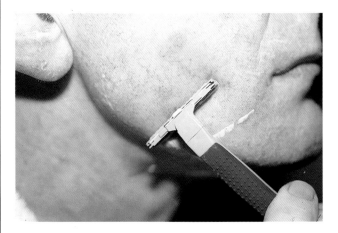

Shaving traumatises the skin – yet it is said that the average man spends six months of his life shaving!

Well-formulated skin care products can help to reduce the discomfort of shaving.

Pre-shaving products

The most important component in shaving, whether with an electric or a manual razor, is the preparation of the skin and beard. Thorough preparation allows the razor to slide smoothly over the skin and minimises damage to the skin surface.

Pre-shave lotions are for use before shaving with an electric razor. They consist essentially of a mixture of alcohol and water together with a small amount of oil to lubricate the skin so that the shaver glides over it easily and irritation is minimised. They also contain astringents.

In wet shaving, the aim is to soften and engorge the beard with water so that the hairs offer the least possible resistance to the blade

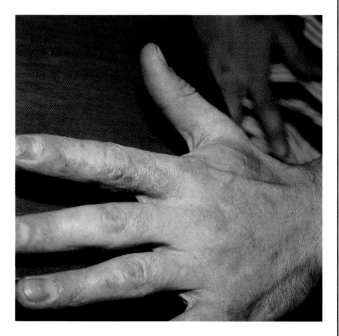

Hand eczema is relatively common among men who do manual work, and should not be neglected.

and avoid trauma to the skin. Washing with hot water and soap before applying a shaving preparation makes wet shaving easier.

Shaving soaps and creams

Shaving products contain soaps, syndets and lubricants. Soaps for the beard are not washing soaps. They are more greasy, and they lather to form a more absorbent, long-lasting, non-drying compact foam which holds the hairs upright, making it easier for the blade to pass through them.

Shaving creams, sometimes called brushless creams, provide a better lubricating action than foams do. Foaming shaving creams are very soapy emulsions consisting of 40–50% fatty acids. Aerosol shaving creams contain soaps that are very soluble in water, presented ready-foamed as they leave the aerosol can by the pressurised gases in the packaging.

Aftershave products

Aftershave lotions are mixtures of similar ingredients as those in pre-shave lotions. The alcohol they contain removes the last traces of cream, the astringents close the pores in the skin (left wide open by the hot water), and a small amount of antiseptic acts as protection against infection of any tiny cuts or scrapes made by the razor.

Moisturisers

Regular use of a well-formulated moisturiser is to be encouraged, if only because of the daily trauma inflicted on the skin by shaving.

More men are also recognising that for long-term photoprotection it is sensible to use a moisturiser that contains a sunscreen, and to use it regularly.

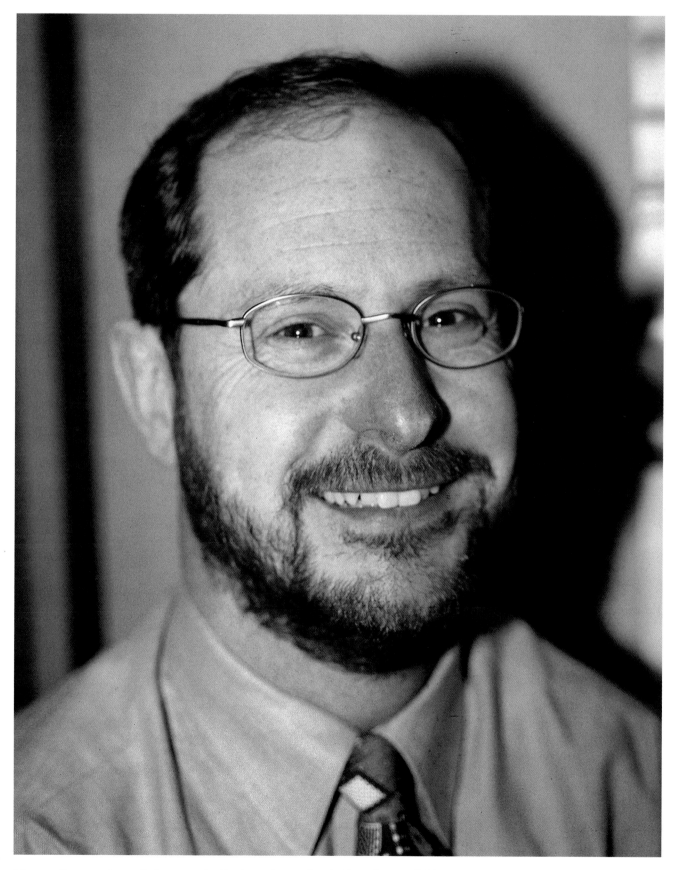

Many well-groomed men today recognise the importance of protection of exposed skin.

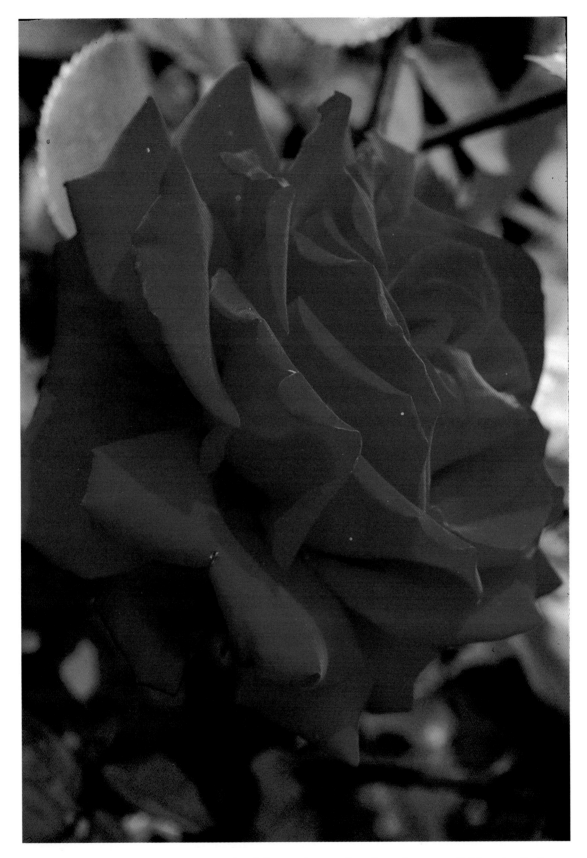

The rose has been one of the world's best-loved flowers since ancient times, its unequalled beauty of colour and form being complemented by its wonderful fragrance.

9

Fragrances

Fragrances have been used throughout history, and were probably in use before recorded history began. Records going back for thousands of years show that wealthy and powerful women used natural perfumes obtained from plants and animals as subtle agents of seduction. In ancient Egypt, strongly perfumed extracts of spices were used in the embalming of the dead. The early Romans were fond of using rose water, and the streets of ancient Rome were lined with shops selling perfumes.

Although not strictly a part of skin care, fragrances are intimately associated with skin.

The sense of smell

Smell is one of the most powerful senses present in all mammals, including humans. It helps protect us from danger and helps locate food. Throughout the animal kingdom, the sense of smell plays a significant part in the search for a mate.

People's ability to perceive both strong and subtle odours varies widely, and depends in part on both sex and age. Women are believed to have a more sensitive sense of smell than men, and have the highest sensitivity from their mid-twenties to the mid-thirties. Many individuals find that their sense of smell becomes less acute as they grow older.

As far as humans are concerned, about 400,000 chemicals have odours: some odours are found pleasant by most people, others are not. The words 'fragrance' and 'perfume' are generally used to describe pleasant smells, whereas the word 'smell' is a neutral term used to describe both pleasant and unpleasant odours.

Fragrances and cosmetics

The relevance of fragrances to skin care is that they are added to both skin care and cosmetic products in order to give these a satisfying scent, thereby making people who use them feel more attractive. On the whole, similar fragrances are used throughout the range of a brand of body care products.

Some cosmetic ingredients have disagreeable odours, which can be masked by adding perfumes to make the product acceptable. Smell is also one of the first characteristics of the cosmetic that the consumer experiences and may become vital to the success of the brand.

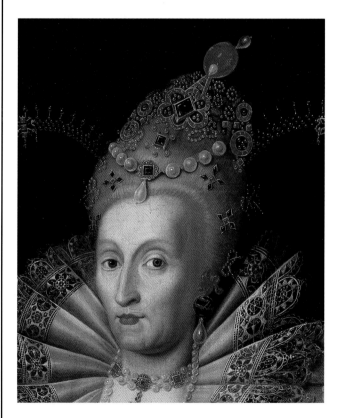

At the royal court in Tudor days 'sweet breath' was prized as much as facial beauty, and perfumes were highly valued in a society where few people paid much attention to washing.

Perfumery raw materials

The classical raw materials for perfumery can be divided into four classes:

- oils extracted from plants
- extracts from animal glands
- chemicals isolated from natural perfumes
- synthetic chemicals produced by chemical reactions.

Natural perfumes

Natural perfumes are complex mixtures of substances. Extracts of the flower jasmine, for example, form part of many commercial perfumes and have more than 200 components. These range from jasmine lactone, with a pleasant smell, to indole which when pure smells extremely unpleasant but which when present in only tiny amounts has a floral scent; the scent of the mixture as a whole is beautiful.

Natural perfumes are obtained from plants by separation procedures such as distillation. They are mostly oily materials, and may be extracted from flowers, fruits, seeds, woods, branches and leaves, bark or roots. Flower scents have been popular among people of every period and culture. The most important of these scents are rose, jasmine, muguet (lily of the valley), lilac, carnation, tuberose, hyacinth, orange blossom, violet, heliotrope, gardenia, honeysuckle, jonquil, narcissus, freesia, ylang ylang (an aromatic Asian tree with yellow flowers) and daphne.

Natural extracts from the scent glands of animals such as the musk deer and the civet cat were used for centuries as perfume components.

Musk was once the most important perfumery raw material. It has always been difficult to obtain and extremely expensive, since the male musk deer from which it is derived lives in remote and mountainous regions.

The musk deer is now extremely rare and the civet cat is extinct. Nevertheless the perfume industry has developed chemicals that have the same scents as the extracts from the bodies of these animals, but which can be synthesised in large amounts comparatively cheaply, and these are now widely used.

Aroma chemicals

The demand for perfumes has increased throughout the twentieth century, and synthetic **aroma chemicals** have come to dominate the market. The term is used for single chemicals of known molecular structure.

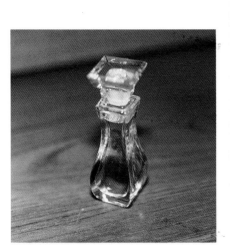

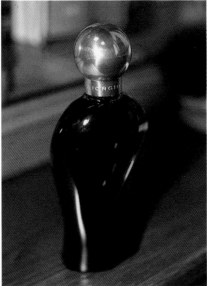

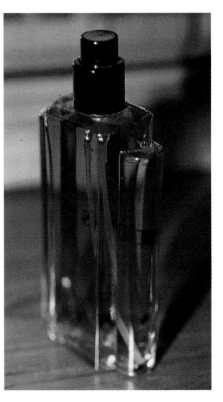

Many are identical with the constituents of natural perfumes but in addition, new chemicals with good smells not found in nature have been synthesised, and expectations for aroma chemicals are growing steadily.

Fragrance compounds

The process of imparting a fragrance to cosmetics is called **perfuming**. The natural perfumes and aroma chemicals described above are rarely used on their own; they are nearly always blended together for some specific purpose. Such blends of natural and synthetic substances are called **fragrance compounds**.

Perfume creation

The expert who creates perfumes for alcoholic fragrances and cosmetics is called a **perfumer**.

The perfumer can select from about 500 natural aromatic raw materials and 1000 aroma chemicals, blending them together to create a perfume matching the required image. Simple perfumes may contain a blend of 10–30 materials whereas complex sophisticated perfumes may contain 50–100 substances. In the most extreme case, many hundreds of materials may be blended together to suit a particular purpose.

Different fragrances tend to be used in different types of cosmetics. Generally popular fragrances such as rose, jasmine, lily of the valley and lilac are used for lotions and creams. For make-up cosmetics, powdery and sweet fragrances have been widely used, but recently floral fragrances have become more popular. Overall, there is a trend towards subtle and sophisticated fragrances.

Men and women have different preferences for the strength of a fragrance, but at the same time, the fragrance is used to appeal to the opposite sex.

The International Fragrance Association (IFRA) has determined guidelines for safe use of perfume ingredients, which are followed worldwide by the manufacturers of cosmetic fragrances. In addition, a large amount of research is being conducted into new and existing perfumery materials to ensure safe marketing for consumers.

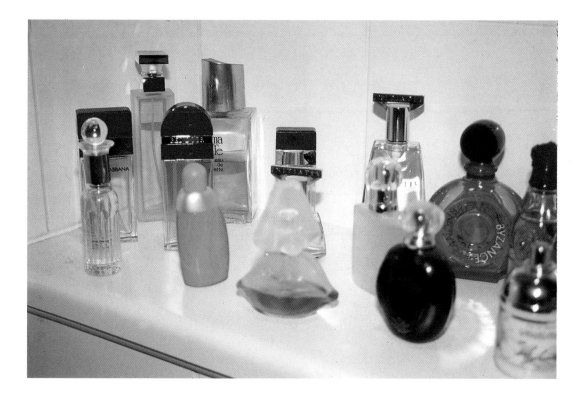

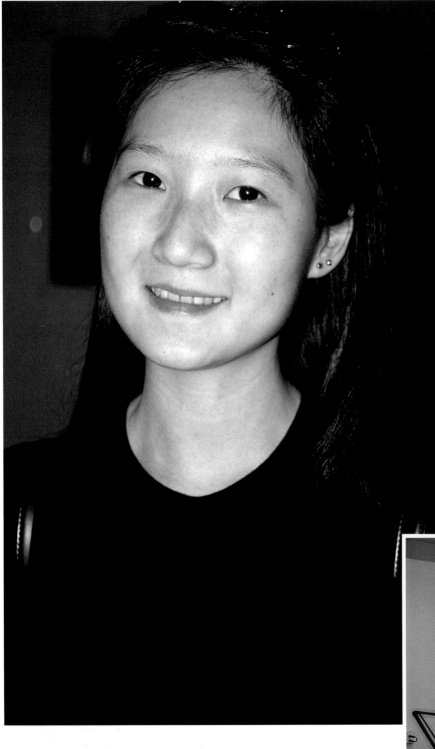

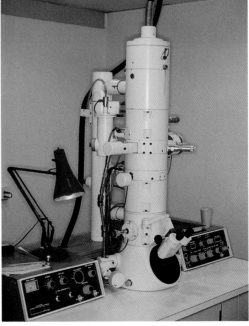

Confidence – backed by the science that underlies cosmetic products.

10
The safety of cosmetic products

Millions of people use cosmetic products regularly, and many of them use several products daily. Yet few ever stop to think of all the research that went into their development, testing and manufacture.

We all rely on our cleanser, moisturiser, make-up and perfume to deliver consistent results, and trust their manufacturers to ensure that their products do us no harm.

In this chapter we outline the type of testing that the cosmetics industry puts into ensuring that their products are safe, effective and reliable.

Methods for evaluating skin characteristics

For a long time scientists believed that intact skin formed an impenetrable barrier through which chemicals could not pass. Compared with most other tissues, the skin surface is only slightly permeable. But nearly all substances do eventually penetrate skin to some extent and finally enter into the blood or lymphatic vessels. Whether a given substance is easily absorbed depends in part on its physical and chemical properties: compounds that penetrate most rapidly and deeply generally have fairly small molecules. It also depends on the composition of the product, particularly on what is called the **vehicle** – an inactive substance that is mixed with the active ingredient(s) to give bulk. For instance, lotions are more active than gels in aiding ingredients to penetrate the skin barrier.

When a cosmetic is applied to the skin, all its components can be absorbed by the skin to some extent, with effects that may (or sometimes may not) benefit the user. On this basis rest cosmetic manufacturers' claims regarding skin moisturisation, smoothness, suppleness and hypoallergenicity.

The cosmetics industry concentrates much effort on using modern technology for investigating the validity of these claims, and also for studying how cosmetic products affect the skin. The need to obtain scientific data to prove advertising claims has led to an enormous development in instrumentation designed to examine in detail minute differences and changes in skin.

Measurements are made of the following features of skin, which both highlight the differences between skin types and which also can be used to measure the results of using different skin care products:

■ skin surface appearance
■ stratum corneum hydration and
■ sebum secretion.

An individual's skin, as we have seen, varies from one part of the body to another. Moreover, there are great variations in the skin of different individuals. It is usual therefore to measure the changes in a single feature of one skin area on one particular individual. For example, the appearance of dry skin before treatment may be compared with its appearance after one, two or three weeks of, say, moisturiser or steroid application.

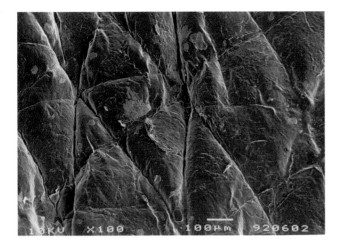

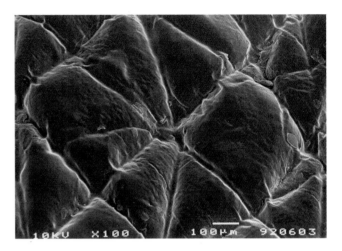

An electron microscope, shown on page 136, can achieve a far higher magnification than with an ordinary microscope; here the electron microscope 'sees' the skin surface (left) before and (right) after treatment with a skin care product, showing how the dead squames have been smoothed down.

Study of skin surface appearance

Skin surface relief
The first step in all methods for studying skin surface relief is the preparation of a replica of the skin surface in three dimensions to an accuracy of less than 1/1000 of a millimetre, using silicone polymers. This is followed by scanning at high magnification so that tiny irregularities on the surface can be observed and recorded. The reconstruction allows scientists to measure certain characteristics of roughness.

Repeating this process by making numerous scans over the whole area enables the skin surface to be reconstructed and its average characteristics determined.

Recent improvements have replaced the mechanical scanning used in the original instruments with optical scanning by means of laser beams (**laser profilometry**). This is an extremely sophisticated technique, however, and available in only a few centres. Another approach involves digitisation of an image of the replica, which does away with the need for cumbersome and expensive equipment.

Skin surface relief studies can demonstrate changes in the amount of wrinkling and in the state of hydration of the stratum corneum. An increase in hydration amounts to an increase in swelling (turgor) of the cells, seen as a smoothing out of the relief.

Skin surface biopsies
A skin surface biopsy consists of taking a small sample of the stratum corneum. It is a simple, non-invasive and painless technique, which can be done in two ways.

The first uses cyanoacrylate glue spread on to a flexible plastic slide, which is applied firmly to the skin for about 30 seconds. Removal of the slide after this time detaches between three and five layers of corneocytes.

In the second method small, transparent adhesive discs are used to remove the corneocytes.

Whatever the technique used, the samples of cells can be stained (to make the features of the cells clearly visible) and examined with a microscope. The images obtained can illustrate various states of the skin surface.

Skin hydration measurements

When a manufacturer is considering the formulation of a moisturiser, it is useful to be able to measure any change in stratum corneum hydration induced by the new product.

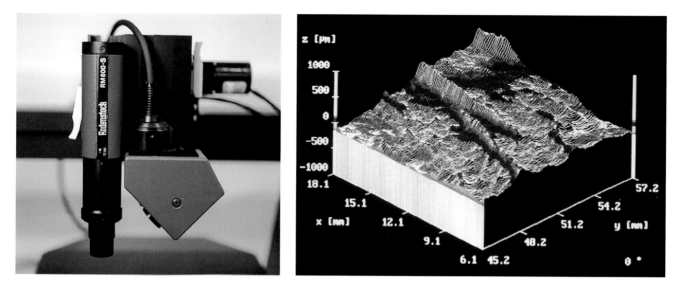

(Left) A laser profilometer, which can produce (right) an accurate computer-generated image of the skin surface.

One technique relies on the indirect measurement of electrical capacitance (strongly influenced by water content). Another measures the rate of transepidermal water loss (TEWL) (water loss by evaporation from the skin surface), and another the surface tension of the skin.

The corneometer
The dielectric constants of keratin and lipids are very small compared with that of water. (The **dielectric constant** of a material is a number that reflects the electrical properties of that material.) Therefore the dielectric constant of the stratum corneum is determined by its level of hydration: the greater the water content, the larger the dielectric constant.

The **corneometer** is an apparatus that uses this relationship. It carries a probe that is placed in contact with the skin. The probe acts as a capacitor, which is a device for storing electrical charge. Its capacitance is proportional to the dielectric constant of the skin, and varies according to its state of hydration. It is possible to distinguish between dehydrated skin, skin with a tendency to dehydration and normal skin using this method. In practice, however, the technique is used to measure the difference in stratum corneum hydration before and after the application of a cosmetic or other skin treatment. The corneometer is both reliable and simple to use.

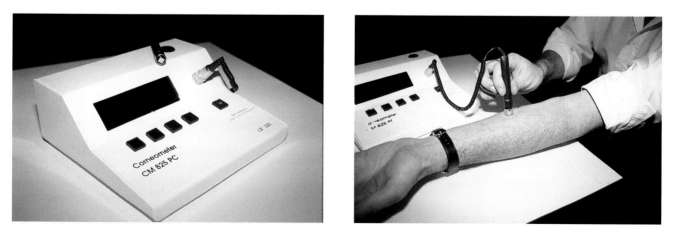

(Left) A corneometer, designed to determine the dielectric constant of the stratum corneum, and hence its water content; (right) the corneometer in use.

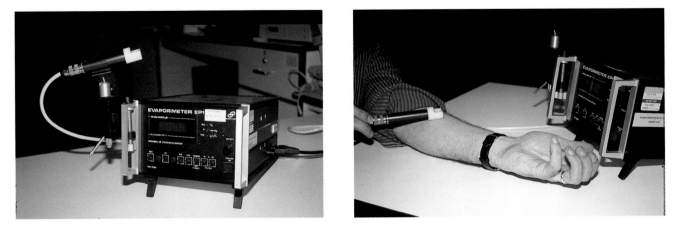

(Left) An evaporimeter, designed to measure transepidermal water loss (TEWL); (right) the evaporimeter in use.

Measurement of transepidermal water loss (TEWL)

Measurement of TEWL uses an instrument called an **evaporimeter** to determine the amount of water vapour that moves across the stratum corneum. It does not measure skin hydration. It does, however, enable scientists to evaluate the effectiveness of moisturising products that rely on occlusion (once the water contained in the product has evaporated). The TEWL will fall with occlusion.

Normal TEWL values are between 2 and 5 g/m² per hour. They can reach values as high as 90–100 g/m² per hour after skin stripping or in the case of eczematous skin.

Sebum measurement

Sebum production is measured using a special opalescent plastic film, which becomes transparent when in contact with sebum lipids.

The device relies on a probe that presses a piece of the special film (renewed for each measurement) on the skin for a measured length of time. The sebum lipids are adsorbed on this film (like ink on blotting paper) and it becomes more or less transparent. The probe is then placed into a device that shines a light beam on to the film. A metal mirror behind the film reflects the beam back again through the film, and then into an instrument called

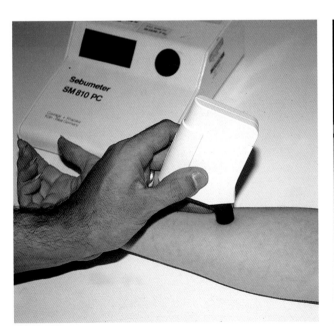

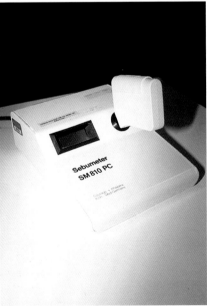

(Left) The probe used to collect a sebum sample, and (right) measuring the amount of sebum collected on the probe.

a photomultiplier, which measures the amount of light in the beam. The more sebum on the skin, the more transparent is the film and so the greater the amount of light reflected.

Regulations for cosmetics

All governments in the developed world lay down controls on the safety aspects of both cosmetics and drugs, in order to protect their citizens.

The distinction between cosmetics and drugs is increasingly important. Each government decides for itself what is a cosmetic and what is a pharmaceutical product, and the decisions can vary from one country to another. The same product (an antiperspirant, say) may be classified as a cosmetic in the European Community (EC), a drug in the United States and a 'quasidrug' (literally, a 'nearly-drug') in Japan.

In the EC the definition of a 'cosmetic product' is much broader than that of a drug. In the USA, on the other hand, the range of 'cosmetics' is smaller, and there is a degree of overlap with the range of 'drugs'.

The safety and benefits of cosmetics are primarily the responsibility of the manufacturer. Within the European Union, however, certain regulations concerning cosmetics have been agreed by many countries. In other countries there are different regulations.

Recently introduced rules – collectively called **the Sixth Amendment to the Cosmetic Directive** of the European Union, and at the time of writing shortly to be amended again – require companies in member states to provide **ingredient labelling** on all products. They are also required to keep a **Product Information File** (PIF) for each product, which includes all available information on the product.

Ingredients in products must be listed on the label in a standard way defined by the *International Nomenclature of Cosmetic Ingredients* (known as the 'INCI list'), which also details the allowable concentration. This list and ingredient concentration is the result of a huge body of risk assessment research by industrial and academic scientists aimed at defining what are 'safe levels' of cosmetics ingredients.

Ingredient labelling follows the INCI nomenclature mentioned above, and enables interested consumers or doctors to identify ingredients. Perfumes, some of which are mixtures containing hundreds of ingredients, are however exempt from the legal requirement to list every single constituent.

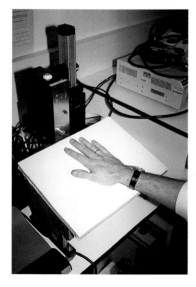

Measuring the surface tension of the skin: this provides an indication of the level of moisturisation in the skin.

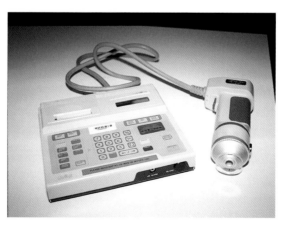

(Above) A colorimeter, an instrument that accurately measures the colour of the skin, which gives information about the blood flow beneath the surface; (right) the colorimeter in use.

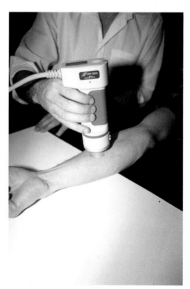

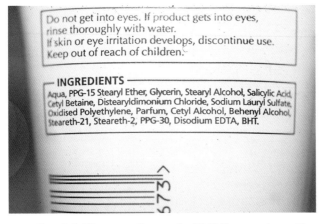

Ingredient labelling according to the INCI list, together with safety notes.

Companies are further required to record any 'undesirable health effects' of marketed products, and to hold those records for inspection if required. The exact definition of such effects is not clear, and has not been established in any court of law. In any case, all reputable companies record all consumer and medical reports and attempt to investigate many of them.

Safety of cosmetics

Every year, manufacturers spend millions of pounds examining ingredients that they are considering using in cosmetic products.

Many of these ingredients have been used for decades and are known to be very safe. For instance, the glycerol used in moisturisers brings significant benefit, does not cause allergies and is very mild to the skin.

Some 9000 ingredients are available for use in cosmetics. The chemistry of these has been studied in great detail to ensure they are safe in the probable conditions of use, and even of misuse as far as this is foreseeable.

It is rare for a brand-new ingredient to be incorporated in cosmetic products. When this is proposed, the ingredient must be subjected to exhaustive examination. In many countries the procedures to be used are laid down in detail by the government.

Most cosmetic products are manufactured from ingredients that are included in a published standard list (for instance, the

European Inventory of Existing Chemical Substances). Substances on this list and others like it have been approved by governments world-wide.

All cosmetics are combinations of ingredients, however. Very occasionally ingredients that are perfectly safe in themselves may interact to produce effects that might possibly be harmful to a few users. New combinations of ingredients – even when all their components are well known – are therefore routinely tested in just the same way that a new ingredient is tested. All finished products too are subjected to rigorous safety programs and quality-assured manufacture by major firms, long before being launched on the market.

While cosmetics contribute to beauty they also play a part in health, taking that term in its widest sense including the psychological feeling of well-being that comes with true good health. Many advertising claims emphasise the 'treatment aspect' of products, so people wanting to buy skin care products are expecting their purchases not just to benefit their skin, but to be completely safe in use, that is, to carry no risk at all.

That certainty of safety must of course relate to the use of the product under the recommended and expected conditions of use.

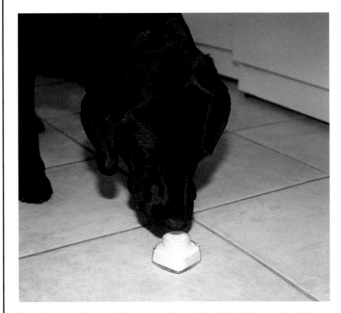

Imminent misuse of a cosmetic product! but the product has been formulated so that there is no risk of any harm coming to the animal

It must equally apply to reasonably foreseeable conditions of misuse: the product might be applied too frequently or on too large an area of skin, or it might even be eaten by a child or pet.

For similar reasons it is important that directions on the packaging are adequate, clearly stated and easy to read.

Safety assessment of cosmetic products

As we have seen, before a cosmetic product is sold it will have been carefully assessed to confirm that it delivers what it promises, and also that it is safe. No responsible company will market the cosmetic until it has been through a process known as **risk assessment**.

This process includes certain tests that scientists may wish to perform, provided they are sure there is no potential for harm. Some of these tests are outlined here.

Pre-launch testing
Preparations of the ingredients under test are placed on the skin of volunteers and kept under occlusion (i.e. covered, with air excluded) for up to 48 hours at a time. They are then reapplied between six and nine times, to see whether they might induce an allergic reaction or cause irritation. The test is repeated with many different people, who between them have every possible type of skin.

This procedure is approved by governments and is very safe, as the scientists who carry it

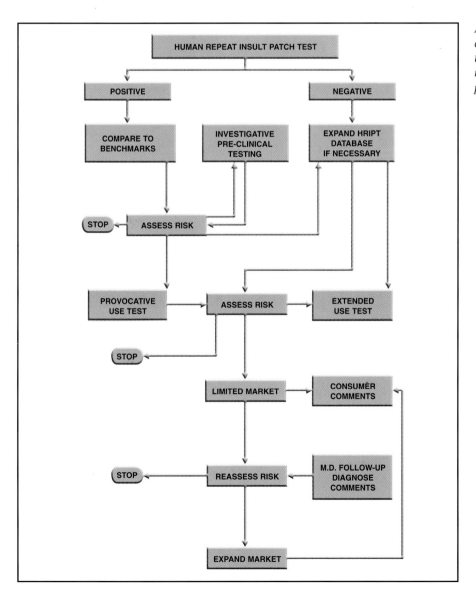

A cosmetics manufacturer follows an elaborate standardised procedure for the full assessment of any risk that may be presented by a proposed new product.

out are extremely careful in determining what concentrations should be used. If the ingredient passes it may be incorporated in a cosmetic, although almost certainly at a much lower concentration than that used in the test.

Sometimes a product that produces few if any allergic reactions in these tests is labelled as 'hypoallergenic'. There is no agreement as to what this word means, however, and it has been banned in some countries because scientists believe it can be misleading.

Percutaneous absorption
In order to predict the activity of the safety of cosmetic ingredients, it is important to measure their rate of penetration into and absorption through the skin. This **percutaneous absorption** can be measured directly, by finding out the amount of a substance under test reaches the lower levels of skin, or the blood in the underlying vessels, within a certain time.

Safety in use testing
This type of test follows the careful assessment of a product based on the ingredients in its formulation. A dermatologist supervises the use of a product in many patients to ensure that even if it is used for several weeks on end, it will not cause any problems to the user.

Post-marketing surveillance
Most major manufacturers ensure they can follow up with consumers or other interested parties any skin problem that may be associated with the use of a cosmetic product.

All product labels must carry the name and address of the company and many have a toll-free telephone number by which they may be contacted if any such problem arises.

Follow-up may include referral to a specialist dermatologist, and patch-testing the product and/or its ingredients to see if it really was responsible for the problem.

For personalised skin care advice, call FREEPHONE 0800 708 708

A product label providing a toll-free telephone number to contact with any query.

Skin problems associated with cosmetics

Considering the millions of products that are sold every year, problems with cosmetics are very rare. The most common cause of those that do occur is skin irritation.

Surveys consistently reveal that up to 70% of all women consider they have sensitive skin. Presumably they think so because they have at some point experienced irritation from, say, a cleansing product that was too harsh.

Modern cleaning products are specially formulated to minimise the risk of irritation, and many include built-in moisturising ingredients.

People with the condition called **atopic eczema** (see page 54) seem especially prone to suffer irritation. This type of skin has a greater than average rate of transepidermal water loss and is unusually susceptibile to harsh surfactants.

Environmental conditions always need to be considered when the causes of skin problems are being investigated. Women in 'wet work', such as cleaners and hairdressers, are by far the most vulnerable group. In agricultural workers, light machinery operators and meat handlers, too, intrinsic skin damage is frequently made worse by not wearing gloves at work.

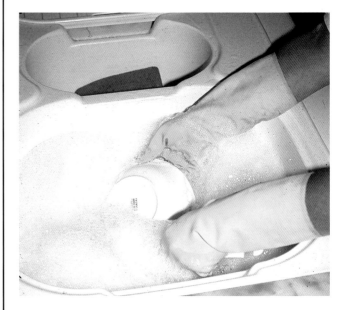

The routine wearing of protective gloves spares the hands from contact with hot water and strong detergents. This is an important part of skin care.

Skin allergy to cosmetics

Sensations of pleasant tingling, or even gentle smarting, that are felt very rapidly after the use of a product such as an aftershave or an astringent are almost normal. They are due to the alcohol content of the product and are *not* allergic reactions.

Genuine allergies to well-manufactured cosmetics are rare. Most of the allergies that do occur are the result of previous repeated encounters with an ingredient in a product with an unsatisfactory formulation. The person becomes **sensitised** to the ingredient, and a later encounter with a very low and perfectly legal concentration of that substance may stimulate an allergic reaction characterised by a rash.

Allergies can only be diagnosed after patch testing by a dermatologist. Most rashes are in fact likely to be slight irritation. The table opposite shows the difference between irritations and genuine allergies.

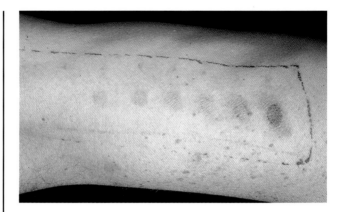

Testing for allergic sensitivity, using progressively more dilute solutions on forearm skin.

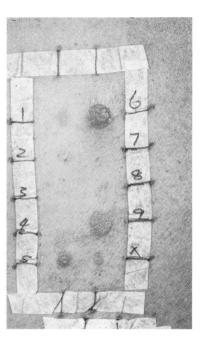

Confirming allergies: the results of a patch test on the skin of a patient's back.

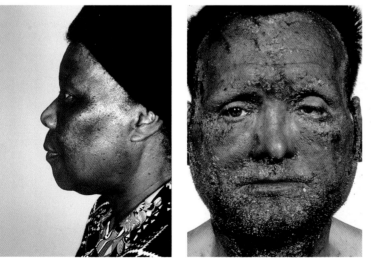

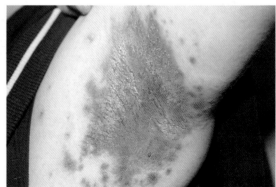

Some rare allergic reactions to cosmetics: (left) to hair dye, (middle) to a beach sunscreen, (right) to a poorly formulated antiperspirant.

Comparison of irritant and allergic contact dermatitis

Feature	Irritant	Allergic
Substances causing problem	Water, soap	Nickel, fragrance, hair dye
Distribution of reaction	Localised	May spread beyond area of first contact and become generalised
Concentration of agent needed to cause reaction	High	Can be minute
Timing of reaction	Immediate to late	Typically 24–72 hours
Immunology	Non-specific	Delayed hypersensitivity reaction
Diagnostic test	None	Patch test
Who is vulnerable?	Everyone	Only a few people

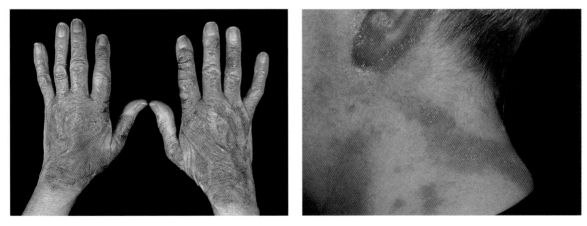

Skin reactions to irritants: (left) irritated skin around the eyes, caused by a poorly formulated cosmetic product, (right) exfoliation of hand skin caused by an irritant cleansing liquid.

Skin allergies: (left) to a plant (primula), (right) to an antibiotic.

And finally...

We hope you have enjoyed reading this book and that it has provided a clear explanation of what skin is, what it does and how we can look after it.

Remember that the way our skin looks is a combination of what we were born with, how long we have lived, how much we have damaged it and how well we looked after it.

The most important messages for a lifetime's care are:

1. **Protect children's skin from the sun**

2. **Teach good skin care from a very young age**

3. **As a teenager, cleanse regularly to keep spots at bay**

4. **As an adult, cleanse regularly with mild products**

5. **Avoid the sun**

6. **Use a daily moisturiser with sunscreen against UVA and UVB, and a night moisturiser as well**

7. **Take extra care of the face and hands**

8. **Well-formulated hydroxy acid products can help to reduce fine lines**

9. **In later years use heavier-duty moisturisers, particularly at night**

10. **Always read the instructions!**

Index